The Purposive Brain

The MIT Press
Cambridge, Massachusetts, and London, England

The Purposive Brain

Ragnar Granit

Acknowledgments

For permission to reproduce figures from a number of publications I
wish to express my gratitude to Acta Physiologica Scandinavica, Journal
of Physiology (London), The Macmillan Company of London and New
York, The Plenum Press, New York, and The Societas Scientiarum
Fennica.

This book was set in V-I-P Baskerville by The MIT Press Media Depart-
ment Computer Composition Group, printed on R & E Book and bound
in Holliston Roxite "B" by the Colonial Press Inc. in the United States of
America.

Library of Congress Cataloging in Publication Data

Granit, Ragnar, 1900–
  The purposive brain.

  Includes bibliographical references and indexes.
  1. Brain. 2. Neurophysiology. 3. Neurophysiology—Philosophy.
    tle. [DNLM: 1. Brain—Physiology. WL102 G759p]
QP376.G69 152.3 77–2347
ISBN 0–262–07069–3

Contents

Preface

Having finished this book, I really feel that the preface should be written by someone less personally engaged in it than myself. Let me therefore summarily state that it is concerned with the nature and limitations of the explanations by which we try to understand the central nervous system acting in response to the environment as an interpreter and as a mover of limbs. Explanations cannot be discussed without representative examples of findings that have to be explained. Most chapters contain some experimental results, but three (6, 7, and 8) are largely experimental though provided with historical introductions. Chapter 10—and to some extent Chapter 9—summarizes and reconsiders much of what has been set out in the rest of the book.

This book was planned and begun during a six months' scholarship at the Fogarty International Center, National Institutes of Health, Bethesda, Maryland, 1971–1972. Its two last chapters were written during a second stay of four months in 1975. In expressing my gratitude for these great privileges, I am also grateful for the enormous resources of the National Medical Library in the immediate vicinity of the Stone House residence, not forgetting the excellent Library of the National Institutes, equally close and its people equally friendly and helpful.

I am indebted to the Rockefeller Foundation for a delightful stay at the Villa Serbelloni, its conference center at Lago di Como, Italy, during which I wrote the difficult Chapter 6.

Finally, I wish to thank my former secretary, Miss Gunvor Larsson, for typing the manuscript.

Ragnar Granit

The Purposive Brain

1
The General Nature
of Biological Explanations

In dealing with objects of our research whose explanation from the standpoint of present-day sciences is insufficient, greater scientific clarity is achieved by fully realizing what cannot be explained than by stealing a march on science with suppositions. We cannot reach farther than to understand what can be understood and realize what we cannot understand. (*The Autobiography of Berzelius*.)[1]

Physics and Biology

The degree of satisfaction that a biologist derives from his explanations depends not only on their completeness and neatness and the terms in which they are couched but also on the preferences and interests of the person. There are those whose appreciation is reserved for mathematical, physical, or chemical explanations, all of which signify that an attempt has been made to incorporate new results or conclusions with a structure of known rules and relations, the great edifice of those sciences. Others are more interested in trying to expand their science by developing a structure of a different kind, one that is exclusively biological, concerned with interpretations of a very different order, aimed at understanding organisms in relation to their environment. All of us are in the end fated to beat our heads against a wall. The sign on it is *ignorabimus*, "we shall never know." My point is merely that the structure of the wall we find in our way also depends on the head that beats it.

Physics at this impenetrable barrier, starting as all sciences from the contents of our sensory messages, has overcome their narrow limits with the aid of the mathematical instrument. In doing so, it has lost in pictorial directness while gaining in precision. Physics cannot explain the magnitudes of the two great and all-important constants, the quantum (h) and the velocity of light (c). It does not understand the nature of gravitational and magnetic forces, to mention but a few examples. The triumphal progress of physics depends on understanding the relations between mathematically defined concepts and units. With their aid it has created an understandable world when faced with the challenge of harmonizing science and reality.

3 Physics and Biology

It is not my intention to deal at any length with the nature of physicochemical explanations. The physicists and chemists have provided us with a host of learned treatises and popular writings. One point I want to emphasize— because it is equally valid for physiology—is that the insight laid down in the concepts and formulas of modern physics in the end is subject to the rigorous test of applicability. The most famous example is Einstein's equation relating energy and mass, $E = mc^2$, which led to the design of atomic piles and of the atomic bomb.

Berzelius's remark implies that one is obliged to arrive at an understanding of what is meant by speaking of explanations. This means to be able to define the terms in which one expresses one's insight. Berzelius—at the beginning of the last century—knew only physicochemical explanations, and what the word meant to him is clear. It signified causalities (relations) found by experimentation, the broad royal road of natural science of the day. Now, after 150 years, many new biological sciences have arisen: physiology, genetics, psychology, and many others. At one time or another many of them have raised hopes of novel kinds of explanations revolutionizing our understanding of living things. A great humanist such as Ernest Renan thought that the then new science of physiology would provide answers to the question of the essence of life, and the many expectations based on the concept of evolution, from Spencer onward, hardly require any further comments. At the moment the geneticists are in the limelight; among them there are those who think that they know the secrets of evolutionary development well enough—"wie es eigentlich gewesen ist"*—to be ready to undertake controlling the fu-

*The well-known postulate of Mommsen that history should explain "what it really was like."

ture of our species despite the fact that all leading workers in this field admit that the course of evolution is unpredictable.

The physicochemical line of approach is often unassailable and also plays a major part in biology. Crick has stated this standpoint in the following manner: "Eventually one may hope to have the whole of biology 'explained' in terms of the level below it, and so on right down to the atomic level. . . . So far everything we have found can be 'explained' without effort in terms of the standard bonds of chemistry—the homopolar chemical bond, the van der Waal attraction between non-bonded atoms, the all-important hydrogen bonds, and so on."[2]

Crick has put the word "explained" within quotation marks, but what is it he has said, with or without them? Essentially that he, like most of us, has been educated to employ the explanatory chemical or physical terms current in his field of research, and that he, again like most of us, can reach far down into the microworld by using them. When following the physicochemical approach in biology we are "walking in our mother's street"—to use a Swedish expression. We get the replies to our questions in terms we have been taught to employ and regard as correct. No quotation marks are needed for the word explanation. Everything is in order and all of us agree on principles.

Some of us may feel a little apprehensive of extravagant claims based on the notion that the "molecular" mode of questioning necessarily is the one most important and most likely to reveal more than any other approach to biological problems. The student of the central nervous system, for instance, is faced with many fundamental questions at a very different level of interpretation. This is what I shall deal with in these essays.

5 Physics and Biology

Quite generally it can be said that the gain in knowledge, as one penetrates into the microworld, is accompanied by losses at other levels of understanding. For example, twenty years of experimentation have provided us with important and quite detailed knowledge about the chemical and physical events at single contact points between neurons, the synapses; the new facts concern the mode of transmission of nerve impulses from one neuron to the next. Yet all these very important facts represent but a minute fraction of the knowledge we need to understand how one makes a gesture with the hand or interprets a complex visual image.

This situation in biology is commonly understood and in recent years often emphasized, especially by Paul Weiss, who in several books has pointed out the one-sidedness of what is often called a "reductionist" attitude to biology.[3] Weiss has given numerous well-chosen examples of the significance of hierarchical order at the cellular level (see also Hughlings Jackson).[4] This problem turns up with different aspects to physicists among our contemporaries. One way of stating the physicist view is that "complex aggregates of matter generate their own new laws" (Philip Anderson),[5] and Platt[6] has listed the new properties that follow with an increase of complexity of molecules forming lengthening polyatomic chains. Or one might point out that in deriving the gas law by statistical considerations based on the movements of molecules possessing three degrees of freedom, it is not only unknown but also utterly irrelevant how an individual molecule actually has behaved. There is a pragmatic side to science teaching us what can be safely left out. And so it follows that the "machinery" operating nervous transmission at a synapse, while always required to do its job, may or may not turn out to be of much interest for attempts at understanding our upright stance, communication, or visual imagery.

It is in the macroworld of hierarchically organized systems that the biologist must find another set of independent explanations, try to understand what he wants to explain, and explain what he thinks he has understood. There are those who believe that the science called "cybernetics" provides us with the theoretical structure needed for understanding the central nervous system. I shall deal with this assumption in Chapter 10 and explain why I refuse to become a proselyte to this creed, though acknowledging its usefulness along with other approaches to the physiology of nervous events.

Purposiveness in Evolution

In looking for principles, one should begin with some references to what is known about the evolution of beings who have to eat, reproduce, defend themselves, and communicate—things that no physicist need be concerned about. In this field of inquiry one known general principle has universal validity, the idea of natural selection producing adaptations to these challenges of the environment. So important is this principle that by its aid the incisive discovery of the code by which genes are reduplicated, for which Crick, Watson, and Wilkins received the Nobel Prize in 1962, is elevated to a higher level of significance than it could have reached as an isolated discovery.[7] As it is, the mechanism plays a fundamental role in the structural totality of evolutionary theory as a stable factor in the stochastic game Nature keeps playing with our some 40,000 genes.

Zoologists prefer the term "directiveness" in speaking of evolution. They hesitate to use the term "purposiveness" because they feel that "purpose" implies "striving after a future goal retained as some kind of image or idea" (Pantin).[8] Mayr proposes the term "teleonomic purposiveness" (after Pittendrigh) to underline the basic contention of the synthetic evolutionary theory that purposeful adaptations are produced by natural selection operating in a population on the phenotype to test the genetic supply.[9] Recently Monod has used the term "teleonomie."[10] I am quite satisfied with "purposiveness" because, as we shall see, many nervous acts definitely have a purpose but otherwise vary in nature from automatism to definite conscious awareness of what is supposed to be achieved. In considering the central nervous system, the essential point is not that one need be aware of the goal but that the act as such is purposive. The classic term is "teleological interpretation" and I intend to stick to it. It means the kind of interpretation in which "why" is a relevant question alongside the "how" of classic natural science.[11] I shall return to a differentiation of this concept from its evolutionary counterpart in Chapter 2.

Darwin began his analysis of the material collected on his journey in the *Beagle* by studying how skillful breeders produced new strains of animals and plants by selection.[12] In these efforts the purpose of the selecting was more or less clearly defined. When later he understood that Nature did something similar by natural selection, this, too, served a purpose, that of producing and retaining traits favorable for survival. In this century we have seen Mendel's rediscovered experimental approach to heredity lead to a definition of the gene, to experimental demonstrations of mutation, recombination, and other processes within the gene pool of a population as a basis for the emergence of novelty, and to the mathematical development of population genetics as a kind of explanation of how purposiveness is achieved. No doubt a key has been found to one of the many doors locking the entry into full understanding of how useful novelties are stamped in. The evolutionary theory offers the outsider a curious Janus face: on the one hand chance is blind in creating mutations; on the other the test for survival of a trait is its purposive adaptation to the environment. By this it is related to and tested in the outside world. As stated, the mechanism of testing is exerted on the phenotype that is embodying the net result of interacting genetic instructions. Because these are polygenetically determined in the sense that genes influence several "characters," it is difficult to reach final conclusions with specific applications.

However, let us take one thing at a time and consider purposiveness as a scientific explanation of an adaptation. One of the oldest and best known examples is industrial melanism, the augmentation of dark relative to light varieties of some species of moths in the sooty districts of Birmingham and Manchester.[13] Against the black trees the light moths have fallen an easy prey to the birds while the dark ones have had a better chance of survival. This development in the moths has been followed since 1850. I am told by experts that recent control of air pollution has led to reappearance of the light forms. This classic example fits the theory: the gene concerned can produce dark and light varieties of moths. At least in one species the dark varieties are believed to be more vigorous; the light ones in normal circumstances compensate by their protective coloring. Then, as *deus ex machina*, enters man and debases the value of the camouflage of the light moths by removing its purpose. The dark variety of the gene now provides the better match to the environment. The dark moths survive

because of their double fitness: they are better fitted or
adapted to the environment and produce more numerous
offspring (fitness in the genetic sense).

Before anything was known about the genome as the
substrate of heredity, an observer of the moths in their environment could invoke natural selection by itself as an explanation of *why* the light forms disappeared. Knowledge
of the Mendelian gene was required to explain *how* the
mechanism of the color shift operated. On the other hand,
without the initial why question there would have been no
real understanding of what had happened.

We shall find the latter type of teleological explanation
permeating the explanations of responses of the central
nervous system. This structure, after all, is Nature's greatest invention for enabling organisms to deal competently
with their environment. We cannot imagine a nervous system without a purpose, much as we tend to neglect purposiveness when studying the hardware of chemical and
physical events that are the means of realizing this goal.
"Purpose" in our present context, like natural selection in
evolution, is neither chemical nor physical. It is a point of
view, like relativity or quantum mechanics. Such ideas belong to the architecture of understanding rather than to
the analyzable material of the edifice of experimental science. They explain something and they have practical consequences. Because "purposiveness" belongs to a category
of thinking that deals with biological organisms in their relation to the environment, it is by definition part of the
domain of biology.

If we decide to switch from why questions to how questions, we move into the realm of purely causal explanations. These are often usefully predictive. If we know a
causal chain $a - b$ we also know that b presupposes a. The

universal appeal of rigid causal or statistically valid explanations stems largely from the fact that predictability is essential for control and thus for technical developments. Teleological explanations are often held to be unscientific because they so easily fail to be usefully predictive. I shall take up this question in Chapter 2. In the last instance our attitude to these problems also depends on how one wants to define "scientific understanding." I would think it unjustified to call the synthetic theory of evolution unscientific because of its very obvious deficiencies when it comes to prediction. It embodies deep insight into Nature's secrets and will live with us into the future.

On the other hand, the explanatory value of such a general notion as purposiveness in natural selection should not be overemphasized. Many developments cannot be satisfactorily understood on these lines. Even in the case of melanism, it is not known how a gene capable of producing two colorings has turned up, so to speak, in anticipation of changes in the luminosity of the environment. We can, of course, invent a teleological explanation for it, but even in this science of hindsight there is a limit beyond which it is better to admit that we simply do not know. Geneticists admit this by speaking of "open" genetic instructions, polymorphism, and polygenetically determined characters.[14] Another limit is set by the elements of chance and time, which together have played their roles in environments whose nature we can but vaguely conceive by interpreting geological and paleontological evidence. In addition there must be fundamental unknown factors, some of which will be discovered in due course. The relatively new gene multiplication process is likely to become very important.

There is a serendipitous trait in Nature (open instructions!). Something is begun somewhere in the phylum and after some millions of years is found to be useful for something else. Lucretius (in Chapter 4, *De rerum natura*) pointed out that the tasting tongue preceded speech. The dog uses it for removing superfluous heat from the body. Even in monkeys and apes control of the tongue by mechanisms in the brain has not yet led to the elaboration of speech—excluded also for purely anatomical reasons. These are difficulties, which make one suspect that positive factors concerned with labeling, marking, or "stamping-in" are neglected in evolutionary theory. Such difficulties are well illustrated by what is thought about the transformations of the acousticolateral organ in the evolution of hearing. And with this example I am embarking on my main theme, the central nervous system.[15]

Tufts of hair (cilia) on the skin of very primitive fish are mechanoreceptors likely to respond to vibration. At an early stage these ciliated organs are found enclosed in the lateral line, a kind of tube running superficially enough to be often visible. It extends from the tail to the head. Within the lateral line the cilia still occur in groups, but their free ends are now stuck into a gelatinous mass forming a cupula that swings with the movement of the fluid inside the canal. The cilia are of two kinds, kinocilia and stereocilia. In the lateral canal they still possess vibratory sensitivity, but now the location of the larger and thicker kinocilia toward the head or the tail end of each group provides the fish with directional sensitivity to the flow of fluid in the canal, which can be shown by recording from their nerve fibers. There is excitation, that is, discharge of impulses, when the fluid moves toward a kinocilium and inhibition of the impulse flow to movement of that kinocilium in the opposite direction. We must further assume that there has been parallel development of sense organs, sensory nerves, and projections of these nerves to the fish's brain to make these structural transformations useful. Another step in the evolution of the acousticolateral organ has taken place in fish. The canals on the head have in part migrated into the bony structure, where they have bent round to form three semicircular organs ending in an ampulla. The canals are found to be orientated in the three planes of space. All kinocilia are now in the ampulla, still with their free ends stuck into a gelatinous cupula. The whole system is closed so that the fluid, set in motion by acceleration, will bend the swing-door cupula. Movement toward the ampulla is excitatory; away from it, inhibitory. Thus has been created a sense organ, the familiar vestibularis, responding to angular acceleration in the three planes. This structure is retained in all vertebrates from fish upward; basically it regulates postural movements.

Other portions of the lateral line have formed closed sacs, known in fish as sacculus, utriculus, and lagena. The cupula there has changed into a membrane loaded with crystals, the large conglomerates easily seen in fish called "otoliths." The loaded membrane touching the hairs responds to gravity and so records the position of the head. The cilia have retained their original sensitivity to vibration.

Sacculus and utriculus are carried over to terrestrial animals with only slight modifications, but the third sac, the lagena, begins to wind itself into a spiral in snakes. This line of development is completed in birds and mammals, and the structure is now helical. We know it well as the cochlea, containing the organ of hearing, still employing the principle of hair cells touching a membrane, but it rides on another membrane, the basilaris, which the sound waves influence through the well-known structures of the ear. The lateral line has become superfluous on land, but the vibratory sensitivity of the original tufts of hair is now utilized to place the world of sound at our disposal. This they do at the extraordinary sensitivity for vibratory amplitudes of the order of the diameter of the hydrogen atom.

Again, all this would have been useless without a parallel development of the structures in the brain dealing with the interpretation of these highly differentiated messages. And again we must admit that though all these developments are obviously purposive in their coordination, there is no real understanding of how they have been labeled for interconnection and timed to develop with some degree of synchronization. At this level of precise questioning the synthetic evolutionary theory delivers its answers in the form of postulates.

Even purposiveness begins to look questionable when we think of musicality and musical creativity as the end product of the development of the tufts of hair on the skin of a primitive fish. There is no explanation of the talent that made possible the creation of the Ninth Symphony or the *Marriage of Figaro*. Why has musical creativity turned up at such high levels of excellence? A possible answer is that this talent has proved harmless in the process of natural selection and so has escaped annihilation. We can, of course, supplement this with a number of postulates such as that musicality is polygenetically determined in happy symbiosis with some more useful characters. But in the absence of an unequivocal genetical explanation of musicality, one is obliged to confess to a great deal of ignorance because musical creativity is but one of many similar apparently useless talents. This underlines the words of Berzelius: "We cannot reach farther than to understand what can be understood and realize what we cannot understand."

Thus, to sum up, a teleological explanation facilitates understanding of the origin or existence of some evolutionary changes (adaptations). There are others, indeed, some of the most significant ones, whose interpretation cannot be significantly advanced by teleological arguments. It seems likely that purposiveness has played its role whichever evolutionary change is under consideration, but at a certain level of complexity application of this principle is of little avail to the inquiring mind. We are forced to begin with a large blank check on chance.

The Biological Approach

Purely biological understanding in the sense that the explanations arrived at employ neither physics nor chemistry can lead to insights as penetrating as those of the latter sciences. For biology, medicine may play the role that engineering plays for physics and chemistry, that of providing a touchstone for the conclusions drawn. A case in point is the role of the *Anopheles* mosquito in the transmission of malaria.[16] Another example is the cure of contagious disease. For some 200 years immunology has had triumph after triumph, curing such diseases despite its ignorance about the chemical mechanisms involved. A number of gifted people by accurate experimentation established the rules governing the defense reactions of the body and tested them in experimental and medical praxis. A chemical solution of the problem of specificity of antibodies has been reached today, but Jenner, Pasteur, Behring, Ehrlich, and many others did well without it; they gave the science of immunology its form and content and discovered the specificities of the antibodies that present-day immunochemistry is engaged in explaining (the 1972 Nobel Prize in medicine given to Gerald Edelman and Rodney Porter).[17] The same may be said about the many discoveries concerning the action of hormones. Their effects regarded as rules based on accurate observations were mostly described by purely physiological experimentation long before it became possible to isolate them chemically. In both examples discovery and understanding belonged to the realm of pure biology. The ultimate chemical work of isolating and purifying hormones was then taken over by the chemist who, without the insight acquired by biological experimentation directed by physiologists with their why questions, would never have realized that there was a problem to which he could contribute by his particular methods.

It is quite typical of experimental biology at its best that it creates basic concepts of its own, such as that of a mechanism in some small lymph cells capable of developing highly specific antibodies, and that it then proceeds to close in on the subject by whatever methods are available. Any odd observation may serve as a starting point. The Western world first learned in 1722 from Lady Mary Wortley Montagu[18] of the inoculation against smallpox at the court of the Turkish sultan, long before Jenner started vaccination at the end of that century. The next great development, bacteriology, found its major tool in the microscope. And then followed microchemistry and electron microscopy, leading to isolation and crystallization of virus particles and to the discovery of the role of the gamma globulins in antigen formation.

However, it is not my intention to discuss immunology beyond using it as one example of a conceptual independence in biology capable of standing tests of application as rigorous as that of saving the threatened lives of intricate mammalian organisms including man. Similar issues are raised by the physiology of the hormones. In both cases the responses observed are purposive, but, so to speak, purposive as a matter of course without the teleological viewpoint necessarily much in evidence in the experimental analyses. The questions—like those in physics and chemistry—have dealt with how rather than with why certain experimental observations should be interconnected. In the case of the melanism of the moths, the why of this change of pigmentation proved to be an essential link in its interpretation. Some examples will show that the latter type of teleological understanding plays a similarly creative role in experimental studies of the nervous system, the organ par excellence for dealing purposively with the environment.

Particularly instructive from this point of view are the findings by von Frisch on the compass of the honeybee.[19] In neurological research we often enter the nervous system by way of a sense organ, just as von Frisch did when he showed that the eye of the bee is sensitive to polarized light. We have been taught that light is a wave motion traveling at high velocity in a straight line. Uninterfered with, the waves have no specific orientation around the beam but swing in all directions. By a Nicol prism or a polarizing film the waves can be forced to oscillate in a single plane and the light is then said to be polarized in that, for instance, vertical or horizontal plane. Our eyes do not recognize this. But if a second polarizing prism or film is inserted as a detector into the light beam, it will let through all the light, whose plane of polarization coincides with that of the first polarizer, and nothing at all if turned to polarize at right angles to the latter. Thus an eye can detect the degree of polarization of a light beam by transforming it into degrees of brightness.

The eye of the bee consists of a large number of units, each of which is radially surrounded by eight sensory cells. These cells are differentially polarized to be detectors of different planes of polarization. Because sunlight reflected from the blue sky is naturally polarized, the bee has at its disposal a map of the sky by which to adjust its angle of flight. Only part of the sky must be visible. By defining the nature of the sensory instrument used by the bee for orientation, von Frisch had solved a characteristic biological how problem. The next step would have been an intricate piece of neurophysiological analysis: how does the animal manage to keep the angle of flight constant relative to the visual image selected? General solutions of this problem could be suggested, but von Frisch's intuition took him on another course.

The bees were marked and could be observed through the vertical glass wall of an observation hive. There he saw the returning bees execute a special kind of patterned dance (Schwänzeltanz) in two semicircles whose common diagonal always was danced in the same direction, which indicated the direction of the source of honey to other inmates of the hive. The speed at which this pattern was danced indicated the distance to the source. At 100 m the straight, diagonal portion of the ring dance was repeated 9 to 10 times in 15 minutes, at 1,000 m 4 to 5 times and at 5,000 m only twice in 15 minutes. Needless to say, this is only one cue among others based on color sensitivity and smell. Most interesting is the fact that the dance often was carried out at the vertical plane of the hive so that the learning bees had to transpose this message of information to their own horizontal plane of operation.

Much has been left out in this schematic presentation of the solution of a problem of orientation and communication in an insect. But what has been said should illustrate a very high level of purposive behavior, based on the properties of a measuring instrument (a sense organ) and a cellular organization (a brain) of modest bulk compared with our own, yet capable of inventing and understanding a difficult piece of geodetic geometry, of applying it in the service of communication, and of operating a motor apparatus to its specifications. Questions of how and why have been characteristically intermingled in this work. How is it that the bee can respond to what looks like being a reaction to polarized light? Why do some bees dance in this curious fashion on the wall of the hive? What is its purpose?

The why question is tabooed in physical science but here again it is shown to be decisive in experimental biology, which after all deals with beings that—as I said—have to eat, reproduce, and defend themselves by purposive responses to such challenges. For these reasons replies to why questions may often elevate a trivial observation to the rank of an important scientific generalization. In the present case the *Schwänzeltanz* might well have become one of the innumerable forgotten contributions to the roomy shelf of curios in biology had not von Frisch attempted to unmask its purpose. This made his work a fascinating study of the general problem of communication.

Elsewhere I have given other examples illustrating my thesis. For instance, when rods and cones were discovered in the vertebrate retina, had it not become evident that rods dominated in retinas of night animals and cones in those of daylight animals (Schultze, 1871),[20] this discovery would have remained an observation of but limited consequence. Instead, understanding of its meaning (why) made it a cornerstone in a large body of biological research dealing with the adaptation of the eye to light and darkness, rod vision and cone vision, and the rod-free central fovea of the human retina. "Getting used to the dark," asked Craik, "is it physics, chemistry, or physiology?"[21] One could add psychology to the rest. The reply is that it is one of the many problems of a biological science that by nature is eclectic and has solutions at several levels of understanding. We have seen that there are replies to Craik's question at the level of anatomy, including its microscopic approaches. It strikes us as a photochemical problem when we realize (with Boll and Kühne in the last century) that the rods contain a highly light-sensitive pigment, rhodopsin, for vision at dawn and dusk.[22] Its spectral distribution of sensitivity is known and has been measured several times. This requires a photocell and introduces a little quantum physics because light is absorbed in quanta within the pigment. There are purely chemical problems involved in the process of bleaching of rhodopsin by light and its regeneration in the dark. The physiologist traces the curve of its spectral sensitivity by electrical recording of the magnitude of messages at several cell stations on the way to the brain. Finally the psychologist, employing a conscious "photocell," measures the same curve as a distribution of perceived spectral brightness, using, for instance, the absolute threshold of vision as his index.

It is interesting that the photochemist, the physiologist, and the psychologist all really do obtain the same curve representing the spectral distribution of sensitivity of rhodopsin. When by the middle of the last century psychophysics was developed as a science, scientists used to speak of "psychophysical parallelism." Although this is well represented by the present case, it is not generally demonstrable because sensory information mostly reaches the perceptual stage in a highly edited version. For this reason the old term has gone out of fashion. Physiologists are nowadays more interested in the mechanisms of editing than in the cases for which real parallelism can be found. When it is as well documented as rhodopsin, it is also a perfect example of a biological explanation that is complete in itself, combining in its tripartite way replies to questions from the physical, physiological, and psychological sciences. This synthetic statement means that something fundamental has been understood. From this knowledge as a *point d'appui*, one can go on "vertically" (Weaver)[23] to greater depths of insight into the special mechanisms underlying the light sensitivity of the rods (photochemical, chemical, neural, organizational).

The original question of why there are rods and cones in the retina ramified into several directions that in one way or another are concerned with the differences between daylight and night vision. I shall only mention the fact that rods and cones are connected to vertical and transverse layers of neurons in the retina, which as a structure may be regarded as an outlying little nervous center of its own. The message dispatched to the visual cortical areas in the brain is therefore highly organized, and in getting used to the dark a neural reorganization takes place, slowing down differentiation velocity of its responses by making the retina more capable of summing up the effect of quantum catches within larger excitatory units than those employed in daylight. Many hundred rods may be connected to the same nerve fiber and in addition interconnected in the retina.

This example is our first encounter with the fundamental problem of organization in the neurosciences. I shall return to it with more attention to detail in different connections. This particular problem presented itself in terms of anatomy and physiology with repercussions in psychology. Physics and chemistry have provided important tools in its analysis, but the final understanding we seek is couched in different terms and teleological points of view are an essential part of it.

In his books Paul Weiss refers to specificity and organization as two major unsolved problems in biology.[3] The former was exemplified with immunology in which today science is closer to a solution than anywhere else. We shall encounter both problems also in the physiology of the nervous system. Weiss discusses organization from the standpoint of cell biology, whereas I will consider it in relation to our endeavor to understand the mode of operation of the central nervous system.

Concluding Remarks

Inasmuch as science is the art of acquiring knowledge in such a manner that coherent structures of understanding can be erected on the basis of a critical evaluation of evidence, the biological sciences can point to many achievements of the first order. One often encounters the implicit notion that the ultimate aim of biology must be to explain its findings in terms of physics or chemistry. By discussing relevant examples, I have tried to show that such explanations indeed are important but may be so without ever touching fundamental questions concerning living organisms in their relation to the environment. Impulses, for instance, are alike in all sensory nerve fibers and their genesis is reasonably well understood in physicochemical terms, yet this knowledge does not help us very much to understand their different effects on the senses.

Biology is, as I have emphasized, an eclectic science, aided in seeking structural knowledge by results at different levels of understanding. Anatomy is always in the background, providing keys of its own for understanding organized responses discovered by physiological work. The machinery may be satisfactorily understood as a physiological entity, yet the elements of which it is composed need be and often can be described individually by, say, chemistry and microscopical anatomy joining forces. In this way structures of biological knowledge are created, such as systems of hormones holding the secretion of one another in check by neural secretory or vascular mechanisms. There are hormones whose individual chemical composition and enzymatic control of specific activities are known in great detail. A hormone may in addition have definite psychological effects on the emotional state of an animal. Whatever contributes to the understanding of such organized systems or structures, most of which have to deal with a repertoire of many tasks, parallel and in series, also contributes to the completion of the biological explanation, whereas any one of the partial explanations may be of only modest interest as an isolated fact. In this way biology with its different levels of understanding ultimately emerges as a synthetic science trying to create coherent structural knowledge by interpreting the integrated effects of interacting components.

2
Purpose, Chance, and Causality

Every science that is a science will always have to develop its own peculiar and powerful methods of inference and methods of organizing and structuring its field. It cannot abdicate the search for its own rules and its own symbolic representations of its own empirical conclusions, just on the prospect that, with infinitely elaborate computations and great mathematical insight to pluck out the results, it might some day be quantitatively derivable from some more fundamental discipline. (*J. R. Platt,* Properties of large molecules that go beyond the properties of their chemical subgroups, *J. Theoret. Biol.,* [1961]: 342–358.)

From now on I shall not be concerned with the teleological (or teleonomic) explanations of the adaptations which natural selection is supposed to have created in the manner briefly alluded to in the previous chapter. Knowledge and hypotheses in this field have been well summarized in an array of books and papers (Waddington, Mayr, Dobzhansky). [24] Because no better explanation is available than the synthetic theory of the geneticists, I am resigned to an attitude of mild scepticism as to the completeness of its coverage of matters requiring explanations. Admiring their efforts, I shall regard adaptations as established facts and proceed to consider a different aspect of teleology, one we meet in the central nervous system.

In this field the essential questions of physiologists and psychologists tend to concern a related, yet different concept, that of *adaptability*. This is the glorious climax of evolution: to have created a purposive brain with an incredible degree of adaptability as yet by no means fully explored. The concept of adaptation refers to something else; animals are adapted to heat or cold, to respond to polarized light, to swim, to fly, or to feed on grass, but adaptability shows how perfectly and within what limits the various adaptations operate. Many physiological mechanisms have been drawn into the service of adaptability and these have, partly at least, been the subject of study. We shall be concerned with the manner in which adaptability is organized by the neurons and their synaptic network, how it is reflected in cognition, voluntary movement, sensory interpretation, and posture—in short, with the whole machinery as it serves us in our purposive interactions with the environment. The term purposiveness now acquires a different connotation, liberated as it is from the kind of teleonomic directiveness produced by natural selection modifying a genetic code of instructions.

In the previous chapter it was pointed out that why questions could lead us to discovering adaptations which otherwise might have gone undiscovered or have been regarded as irrelevant curiosities. Such questions also play a role for adaptabilities, but in studying them we go a step further and unashamedly mix how questions with why questions, realizing that mechanisms serving adaptability never can be dissociated from the purpose to which they are adjusted. For this, some relations between purpose, chance, and causality need to be considered.

Purpose, Causality, and Chance

The perfect instrument for realizing adaptability is obviously consciousness, but a large number of automatic adjustments to the environment are also eminently purposeful, and their unexpected consequences may fill us with wonder or even surprise. An example will be given in Chapter 3.

In all cases purposiveness implies anticipation of preferred alternatives in dealing with environmental variables. Clearly, therefore, teleological operations aim at becoming predictive, which is another way of stating that they depend on an evaluation of environmental causes. Everything cannot be predicted in detail, but the brain has chosen a heuristic solution out of this dilemma. It has developed an incredibly large number of possible ways of responding purposively to the environmental variables. The final choice between them is left dependent on prevailing circumstances. More often than not the choice is a wholly automatic process.

This may seem surprising, but the best analogy there is to brain function is obtained from a comparison with the immune system (Jerne, 1973)[25] and uses a similar procedure. The small B-lymphocytes (cells), rather than specializing on certain common diseases, generate an extraordinary number of antibodies. Specialization would have led to a fixed rather than an adaptable adaptation. The latter goal is achieved by the existence of random chemical specificities for pattern recognition, enough to match antibodies to most of the inimical epitopes (small patches on the surface of a protein molecule) that are likely to occur. These fits are remembered by the system, and we know them as immunities for the agents that provoked them (when these attacks referred to diagnosed diseases). In this manner the immune system responds adequately to an enormous variety of signals it learns from experience and remembers the lessons taught by foreign agents. The analogy with it can be carried still further: antibodies may cause excitation or inhibition and the cells of the immuno-system both receive and transmit signals.

If this analogy with the immune system is to be valid, there must be comparable elements of chance by multiplication of possibilities in the brain or else we would actually be the mechanical automaton that Descartes would have made us, had he not rescued the situation by letting in the spirit (l'ame).[26] "We may consider the brain as consisting of a multitude of small units, each with its particular morphological (and presumably functional) features. These units collaborate by way of an immensely rich, complicated and differentiated network of connections, which are very precisely and specifically organized. The anatomical possibilities for (more or less direct) cooperation between various parts of the brain must be almost unlimited" (Brodal,

27 Purpose, Causality, and Chance

1975).[27] In addition, there are widely distributed mutable and hence adaptable connections. The important point is that an extreme precision of wiring, based on somatotopic (localized point-to-point) connections, is responsible for inherited fixed effects, while their very large number in combination with the mutable or plastic connections give chance a chance (see Chapter 3). The central nervous system uses the principles of convergence and divergence. Convergence means that fibers from different sites form contacts (synapses) on the same cell; divergence, that the outgoing fibers of one cell spread in different directions to other cells. At the synapse the incoming or afferent message is transmitted to the next cell by means of an intervening chemical process.[28]

If we could insert a large number of microelectrodes into individual cells in different regions of the brain and have their impulses influence a scintillation counter, we would then see an erratic display of bright flashes representing spontaneous activity. It would not be quite like watching the irregular scintillations from cosmic rays, because between some of the flashes from different sites definite temporal correlations could be established by statistical analysis. But this idealized experiment nevertheless illustrates the natural variations of excitability that occur in an organ containing billions of cells connected by convergent and divergent fibers.

Convergence also implies that if one volley of impulses is incapable of discharging a cell, it may yet have been capable of influencing its membrane in the direction of increased excitability. The cell would then be ready to discharge to a subsequent subthreshold array of impulses from elsewhere. This kind of variable excitability expresses itself also in the fluctuations of size and frequency of membrane potentials recordable from the surface of the brain or even from the scalp (the electroencephalogram of Berger).[28]

I have simplified reasoning by merely mentioning excitation, but inhibitory pathways are just as important though often more localized in their distribution. The impulses do not differ in the two cases. They are messages. The excitatory or inhibitory effect is determined by the subsynaptic membrane site on which they project.[29]

The cellular organization of the brain, faced with Nature's capriciousness, as displayed against a background of basic predictability, has thus solved the problem of adaptability anatomically by an immense multiplication of possibilities on the one hand and strictly somatotopic relationships on the other. The former principle is reminiscent of the apparent wastefulness of plants (and animals) in producing seed (sperms, eggs); the latter, of maintaining genetically fixed relationships calculated to safeguard reproducible causal relations with the environment. The waste is apparent only, because in reality economy is reestablished by the capacity for learning, which gradually cements new associations into blocks of instructions. These, too, are teleologically logical (causal) with respect to the environment and thus replace chance with heavily weighted probabilities. For example, the Pavlov dogs learn to salivate to a tone if during the training period a teleological motivation is introduced in the form of anticipation of a reward (reinforcement). Overlapping or redundant projections will be discussed in Chapter 4.

Practical Teleology

Occasionally one meets with the opinion that teleological

and causal reasoning are diametrically opposed attitudes. Such a view can be upheld only by neglecting the decisive causal role of the environment in modeling the purposive neural demands and responses. Clearly it is often possible and even desirable to neglect purposiveness in studying established neural events from the physicochemical point of view. It may well happen that the purpose for a time disappears into midair like the grin of the Cheshire cat. However, if one then tries to stick the pieces of an explanation together but does it in a telcologically illogical manner, the cat again materializes, now grinning derisively at the bungler who is missing the point. We are in fact dealing with two ways—the why and the how—of approaching the same neural event. These are "by no means mutually exclusive. They supplement one another and blend well" (Granit). [30]

Physiologists brought up to study precise mechanism in purely mechanistic terms tend to be cautious in applying teleological reasoning, while ethologists, used to watching animals, do so freely. It is not much of an exaggeration to call their science "applied teleology."

Writing as a physiologist, my experience is that teleological explanations are serviceable in two specific situations: one is in the planning of an experimental approach, when often a sound idea about the purpose of a mechanism can be very rewarding (see Chapter 3). Many examples can be found in the field of hormonal interaction. Another situation arises when an adaptable neural event, electrophysiological or behavioral, is sufficiently well analyzed to make it possible to predict that its purpose would either be well or badly realized by one or several of a number of alternative hypotheses or models. In actual practice this amounts to a choice between teleologically logical and illogical alternatives or, in less sophisticated language, a choice between what makes sense and what doesn't. A simple example: if the skin of a dog is stimulated by an electrical "bite" until the animal starts a scratch reflex, its leg will be found to reach for the site actually bitten. To assume that the dog would search for the irritating bite in a very different place would be teleologically illogical. Much experience and insight is needed for making sensible use of teleological ideas in analyzing highly complex neural responses.

Complexity of Causes

The fact that purposiveness relates an event causally to the environment by no means implies that we would be able to unravel all causal chains involved. The statistical element previously discussed and past experience as retained in memory may prevent us from arriving at the level of causal insight that characterizes many physical or chemical results of experimentation. This need not worry us too much. Also, statistical explanations in physics can be based on a negligible causal insight into the details of the mechanisms described. Why then should we neurobiologists be expected to do so much better with the, say, 10 or 14 billion cells of the brain? Sommerhoff has made an interesting synthesis of purposiveness and causality, however, without making the particular distinction between established adaptations and adaptabilities that is so important in the study of the central nervous system.[31] But his general trend of argument agrees with the attitude adopted here, one that I believe should be acceptable to most physiologists. Sommerhoff developed his theses mathematically at the hand of an example, the servomechanism by which a gun is made to follow its movable target. As to the role of mathematics, I refer to my introductory quotation (Platt).[6]

Study of the brain is still in an early phase and hardly in
need of much mathematics.

One should remember, too, that "Nature rings her many
changes on a few simple themes. The same expressions
serve for different order of phenomena. The swing of a
pendulum, the flow of a current, the attractions of a mag-
net, the shock of a blow, have their analogues in a fluctu-
ation of trade, a wave of prosperity, a blow to credit, a tide
in the affairs of men" (d'Arcy Thompson).[32] Therefore
much remains to be understood behind the façade of an
equation. Physiological knowledge also serves medicine,
and the physician as a rule is more in need of precise information on physicochemical agents involved than in the
mathematics of some fraction of the total operation.

Knowledge of Results

Of the many different mechanisms drawn into the service
of adaptability, one is particularly important for dealing
with the unexpected, and this is the process of checking
and correcting manipulation of objects by the returning
"knowledge of results" studied so much by the psychologists (Annett).[33] It is familiar from the eye and hand combination that makes man superior in adaptability to all
competing species on this globe.

Knowledge of results is incorporated in the scientific
concept of feedback, which is essential for the understanding of biological processes at all levels from enzymatic regulation in unicellular organisms to hormonal and nervous
control of the mechanisms physiologists deal with in the
laboratory or physicians in the hospital. The corrective
negative feedback of engineering science is now so well
known from innumerable servomechanisms that it tends to

be forgotten that feedback control really is one of Nature's major inventions, familiar to physiologists long before it was conceptualized by Wiener (1947) within the framework of cybernetics, the science of regulation.[34] Some examples will be given to illustrate the two main tasks of negative feedback in nervous regulation (1) to counteract the effect of unknown or unforeseeable variables in the environment, thus serving adapatability by error detection and correction, and (2) to stabilize any process that otherwise might overshoot its intended effect within the living organism and so antagonize its own purpose.

In moving about, for example, we commonly encounter unforeseeable changes of loading of our muscles that respond by changes of tension and extension. Both effects are recorded by appropriate sense organs (measuring instruments) in the tendons and the muscles and reported upward in the nervous system. Extension, by the shortest route through the spinal cord, produces a reflex contraction or shortening of the muscle, the so-called stretch reflex (Liddell and Sherrington).[35] Tension similarly generates a reflex slackening (or inhibition) of the contraction. Hence, in both cases the effects, fed back to the motor executive cells in the spinal cord, oppose the muscular process by which they were elicited. Thus the feedback has a negative sign. In both cases it counteracts unforeseen variables and stabilizes muscular action around a useful degree of contraction. Further neural refinement of this mechanism will be discussed in subsequent chapters.

Other negative feedback mechanisms stabilize the discharge of the motor cells of the spinal cord, and one is of great general interest. The outgoing axon (motor fiber) from each of a number of these cells, the motoneurons, sends a recurrent fiber back into the spinal cord where it branches to intermediate internuncial cells that inhibit the firing of the motoneurons. This inhibitory effect is not strong enough to stop a well-supported discharge, but it prevents the firing rate from reaching high values unsuitable for the contractile properties of the muscle fibers for which the axons are destined. The technical term for this governing mechanism of negative feedback is "recurrent inhibition." Recurrent fibers exist in virtually all nuclei of the central nervous system (Cajal)[36] and so negative feedback emerges as one of the fundamental instruments for regulating the discharge rate by itself. Quantitative studies in terms of firing rates of individual motoneurons have shown that the amount of inhibition is directly proportional to the frequency of the outgoing impulses of a firing cell.[37] By this negative feedback mechanism, strongly supported cells firing at fast rates throw out or suppress the action of feebly firing neighbors.

Nervous inhibition by recurrent fibers is one of Nature's oldest inventions and, like all its ancient discoveries, it is used for a variety of purposes. It has been found by Hartline in the retina of the horseshoe crab (Limulus), in which a discharging cell regulates its own firing rate and that of its neighbors by a direct inhibition whose effect is proportional to its own discharge rate and to the distance from the cell on which the inhibition is exerted. Hartline and Ratliff have analyzed the properties of this system quantitatively and shown how it sharpens the retinal image by contrast.[38] Fossils tell us that the horseshoe crab found its final shape some 500 million years ago. In mammals most recurrent mechanisms have become more elaborated. The returning branches act indirectly, through an internuncial cell, which is subject to convergent influences from elsewhere, with the result that the negative feedback can be thrown in or out or be finely modulated in excitability in response to other requirements, a step up in the degree of adaptability.

Immanent Teleology

This concept has been discredited by a taint of vitalism suggesting knowledge of ultimate causes. Vitalism has been dead for over half a century (although one still finds authors engaged in heaping diatribes on its carcass.) But a condescending attitude to "immanens" as such can hardly be justified. We are after all accustomed to many immanent or ultimate properties of matter that are unexplained. There is immanent gravity and immanent magnetism; why not then immanent purposiveness in the biological realm of knowledge? There is no need for the biologist to hedge from speaking of an immanent teleology in the world being studied. It is but a way of stating that one is dealing with biological processes from this highly pertinent point of view.

3
Exploring Adaptabilities

The dog not only walks but it walks to greet its master. In a word the component from the roof-brain alters the character of the motor act from one of generality of purpose to one of narrowed and specific purpose fitting a specific occasion. The change is just as if the motor act had suddenly become correlated with the finite mind of the moment. (C. S. Sherrington in *Man on His Nature*. London: Macmillan, 1941.)

A systematic analysis of adaptability as such has not been much of a recognized problem in the study of the central nervous system, though numerous papers implicitly deal with mechanisms by which adaptability is achieved. It is interesting for a change to look at some of them in a more general perspective. Such questions have come to the fore lately and are destined to occupy a central place in future research dealing with degrees of pliability to environmental challenges. The largest field requiring exploration is the no-man's-land between Nature and Nurture. So far experimenters have been mainly interested in discovering and describing biological adaptations, regarding them as established functions to be analyzed and quantified. But now, after 150 years of experimentation, insight and methods have reached a degree of maturity that permits investigating physiological mechanisms of adaptability from the developmental point of view as well.

The introductory quotation from Sherrington emphasizes the point raised in Chapter 2, that the conscious brain represents the final stage in the development of our capacity to adjust ourselves to external demands. The dog shares with us some of that talent. An adaptation—the dog walks—has become adaptable by being subjected to cerebral control—it walks to greet its master.

However, to start studying adaptability at that level of questioning is to begin from the end, the top level of dog performance. Pavlov did this when he trained dogs to salivate to a tone by the simple expedient of letting a reward of food in repeated trials succeed the tone. To appreciate the role of purposiveness in creating such conditioned reflexes one need only imagine that the reward had been given before sounding the tone instead of afterward. Perhaps after an excessive number of trials an association might have been established, but not as easily as in Pavlov's well-known version of the experiment. The tone was not essential. The dog could just as well have been trained to salivate to something as abstract as the length of time after a warning signal. Purpose, meaning, motivation, and reinforcement are terms that in different ways show what made sense of the undertaking. Then it becomes another matter that pure associative learning also exists—to the extent that it serves some sensible purpose.

Problems of adaptability assume a different aspect at the cellular level. For instance, can we change a normal response of a single cortical cell (or a number of them) by impressing on them properties at cross-purposes with an ingrained purposive adaptation? This points the way to means of measuring the degree and range of adaptability by its resistance to change. The new and antagonistic environmental challenge is used as a test of the openness of the genetic instructions. The conscious brain behaves as if it had been genetically instructed to be maximally open to environmental modifications.

Adapting to Change of Purpose

A case of failure to adapt is provided by an experiment (Sperry) in which the optic nerve of a frog was cut, the eye bulb turned around by 180° in its socket, and regeneration of the nerve allowed to take place.[39] It was found that by some kind of chemically determined specificity the nerve fibers grew into their original sites in their station in the optic tectum. The result meant that the images of the surgically reversed eye were projected the way they had been before the operation and that they were misdirected with reference to the postoperative orientation of the eye bulb.

Although the animal might have been expected to adjust itself to the dislocation of the image, it never did. A fly in the upper field of vision excited the frog to catch it in the lower field. Once established, the ingrained adaptation was too resistant to allow any adaptability.

This experiment reveals inherently open genetic instructions that have been closed—almost certainly by a chemical marker—but it can be shown that originally they were open in the early stage of amphibian development.[40] If at that stage the eye was experimentally rotated (Jacobson), a normal purposive visual reflex arose.[41] Jacobson's analysis (with Hunt) showed the critical period for the operative rotation of the bulb to be between 32 and 40 hours of amphibian life, the retinal ganglion cells being born at about 34 hours and their nerve fibers reaching the optic tectum 15 hours later. Some—ultimately chemical—processes sanctioned by purposive function then operated to close the genetic instructions for good.

Kittens have a postnatal period of optimum adaptability lasting between 24 and 36 days (Hubel and Wiesel).[42] Two independent experiments by Hirsch and Spinelli, and Blakemore illustrate this in a new and interesting manner.[43] They presuppose knowledge of the discovery of Hubel and Wiesel that single cells in the striate visual cortex of the cat are sensitive to the orientation of oblongs or lines shown to the eye within the retinal receptive field of the particular cortical cell that has been isolated for recording by a microelectrode.[44] In the cat an assembly of such cortical cells in the striate visual cortex represents orientations of visual stimuli in a nonpreferential manner. I shall describe the new experiment in Blakemore's version.

Young kittens are provided with a stiff collar that checks head movements and then reared in a vertically or horizontally striped environment. The individual cortical cells adapt to the new environment and now respond preferentially to the direction to which they have been exposed. Blakemore's finding is rather exciting—that no more than an hour's exposure to such visual experiences suffices to modify the preferred orientation of most cellular units in the kitten's striate cortex, provided that this is followed by a minimum of two weeks in the dark. But if the kittens had had more than five hours of such abnormal experience, the effect became virtually ineradicable by other visual stimuli. Nothing else distinguished these cortical units from normal ones. For a modification of this experiment by Maffei and Fiorentini, see Chapter 6, section on contrast and spatial frequency.[110]

What about ourselves? Prisms, inversion spectacles, or even colored filters have been used in a very large number of experiments to create a visual world at cross-purposes with the one ingrained by prewiring and experience in combination. The oldest experiment was carried out by Stratton (1896).[45] "Stratton studied vision without inversion of (the normally inverted) retinal image. The experiments were done monocularly with an inversion lens, the other eye being covered. He wore this lens for eight consecutive days. Physiologically this amounted to a blatant clash between the information from the sensory fields representing the body (surface, muscle, joints, etc.) and those organized to deal with visual space, in which now [the picture was upside down]. . . . On the second day of his experiment the room was upside down but the body was represented in preexperimental terms and was felt as a standard. . . . On the fifth day the new visual space had established itself so well that there was no anticipatory drawing in of the chin and chest when a solid object passed through the visual field in the direction which in normal vision would have meant a blow." [46] Thus the perceived world as well as the reflex motor response to it had adapted to the new experience at cross-purposes with the old one. From work on monkeys we are entitled to conclude that directionally sensitive cells exist also in our own visual cortex. An average response of such cells can actually be studied objectively by measuring the amplitude of electrical potentials evoked on the scalp in response to visual stimuli of variable orientation (Chapter 6). Vertical and horizontal targets are better resolved by our eye than oblique patterns, and evoked potentials by their amplitude indicate these preferential sensitivities.

Maffei and Fiorentini investigated what happened when seven adult subjects wore tilting prisms continually for seven days. The prisms produced a tilt of the target of 30° or 40° from the vertical, and the angle between the apparent vertical and the real vertical was measured and compared with the amplitudes of their evoked potentials to find the degree of perceptual compensation. Perceptual adaptation to the tilt occurred in all subjects in the first hours, and compensation was virtually complete on the second day. The adaptive effects were accompanied by a decrease of the mean difference between the amplitudes of evoked potentials for the vertical and oblique patterns. [47] One component of this faculty was localized by the outcome of this experiment to the sensory apparatus at some point between the retina and the cortical visual area. We are no more conscious of adjusting for a new criterion of verticality than the kitten or the tadpole in comparable experiments. The perceptual net result of all the silent ongoings comes as a surprise.

The open instructions in these examples worked well

enough for the tadpole and the kitten but not for the frog or the cat. There must be some basic difference between cat and man to make us capable of "repurposing" against an ingrained purpose. At least one reason for our greater adaptability can be discerned—the greater complexity of our wiring diagrams. It is difficult to quantify this statement with figures because no methods are as yet available for measuring connectivity. Some figures can be given merely to indicate its nature. Cragg has made a rough estimate from his own work and concluded that 56 neurons are interconnected with each neuron in the monkey visual cortex and 600 in its motor cortex. On his own data these are minimal values, yet they represent a connectivity in excess of that in any manmade computer.[48] The average number of synapses on a cortical cell is of the order of 30,000. There are about 50 million cells per cubic centimeter in the human visual cortex, as against 10 million in the motor field, which has larger neurons. For the cat visual cortex Sholl found the territory of the branches of one neuron (stellate type) to spread within reach of 4,000 other neurons.[49] We do not know the full relevance of the enormous figures for synaptic densities, up to 60,000 on large cortical cells (Cragg). Recent work by Marotte and Mark has shown that normal looking synapses can be inactive;[50] however, these are synapses projecting on muscle fibers. His results, though not convincingly proved, raise the idea that neuronal adaptability may be based also on activation and deactivation of preexistent projections. If neurons really keep a reserve of passive synapses in preparation for various emergencies, this would further extend the likeness to adaptability in the immune system.

For the moment let us remain with the general notion of superabundance of linkages and greater redundancy as the main distinction between our very much larger cortex and that of the cat and begin by considering the question of repurposing in organizational terms. Basically the desired neural organization can be described as an error-detecting mechanism capable of feeding back its information to the perceptive process. The visual perception of the distorted verticality is an illusion, but an important one, as very much of our sensory input is entering through our 2 million fibers in the optic nerves. In the experiments, on the other hand, powerful messages from other sources contradicted it, gravity being particularly relevant. Impulses from the vestibular organs record balance and head position, and sense organs in the ligaments and muscles of the neck support them. Furthermore, sense organs in the soles of the feet, legs, joints, and around the spine record any deviation from the responses required by the existence of gravity. Their presence is reflected in Stratton's description of his experiences as well as in an observation Kohler made while looking at a pendulum through inversion lenses: it swung upside down, but reverted to normal as soon as he touched its fixed end to swing it himself. [51]

Adaptability to prismatic goggles has lately excited much interest. A decisive experiment favoring error correction by feedback was carried out by Held and Hein when they demonstrated that an animal must be allowed to move about and see the deviations from normality reflected in its own movements to be able to correct for the visual distortion.[52] Moved about passively, it fails to adjust to the prismatically induced displacements. Man is likely to do better on purely sensory information, as shown by the experiments by Maffei and Fiorentini.

In following up one series of experiments in vision from frog to man, I have neglected much work on developmental aspects of adaptability that is necessary for filling out the picture. Thus, for instance, the greater plasticity of the developing nervous system is found throughout the vertebrate kingdom. Man is no exception. It is known that if Wernicke's area in the left hemisphere of the brain responsible for comprehending language is destroyed in a child below about age 12, the right hemisphere takes over and full restoration ensues.[53] Later destructions of that same region leave a child incapacitated forever.

This of course raises the question of why another talent, readjusting to visual verticality, is retained in adults. I would like to link the answer with an attractive hypothesis by Jacobson. What I have called the closing of originally open genetic instructions, he speaks of as "specification" of originally unspecified connections. In Jacobson's theory "some neurons are highly specified and all their connec tions are fully determined, but there are also some incompletely specified neurons with indeterminate connections" (p. 333). The early developing neurons tend to be large, with long axons. They form the primary afferents, are somatotopically organized and specified at an early date in embryonic development, and later on are unmodifiable. The unspecified neurons, retaining the property of openness, are small interneurons of various kinds. They have short axons, variable connectivity, and develop later—even postnatally in some parts of the brain. In contrast to the former type, they require stimulation for their development and for maintenance of their function.

In this view the visual cortex of man should be characterized by an abundance of small interneurons with short axons, which indeed is the case. On the whole the great expansion of our cortex, the "roof brain," is an expansion in terms of interneurons. And when I said that the conscious

brain behaves as if it had been genetically instructed to be
maximally open to environmental modifications, the cellular substrate realizing this property is its bulk of unspecified small cells with short axons, long known as Golgi type
II cells. These cells correspond to the small B-lymphocytes
in the immune system, numerous enough to take a chance
on chance and to remember what they did.

Chemical Specification by Motor Neurons

To most of us, everything sensory invading consciousness
is always more interesting than a motor act. But the understanding of adaptability in chemical terms is at a more advanced level in the motor field in which we deal with long
axons (motor nerve fibers) and synapses accessible in the
muscles they innervate. Even if we do not fully understand
how chemically traceable modifications in muscles are
brought about, the road of advance has been opened. The
adaptability to be discussed concerns muscle fibers influenced by their motor axons. Each axon divides to innervate
a large number of muscle fibers. The motor cell (or motoneuron) *plus* its axon *plus* the muscle fibers that the axonal
branches innervate by synapses is known by the technical
term "motor unit."

With regard to environmental factors, muscles, like so
many other tissues, show a general adaptability to use and
disuse but are stable in their organization. Thirty years ago
Sperry surgically cross-united nerves to antagonistic muscles in rats and monkeys and found a persistent lack of adaptation to the reversed tasks.[54] Even in young animals the
reflexes failed to become reorganized, in rats not at all, and
in monkeys with notable deficiencies.

Contrary to this experience, neurosurgeons operating to

restore lost function in disabled limbs of patients report that any muscle and tendon in the hand and the forearm, when transferred to a new site, can carry out any desired motion. Thus, in *Bunnell's Surgery of the Hand* it is stated that "a wrist extensor can act as a digital extensor, a digital flexor, a wrist flexor or a motor for opposition and adduction of the thumb."[55] As with adaptation to verticality, here, too, our internal computer seems to be of a superior type. But repurposing has to be checked by internal feedback, within the brain itself, as well as by external feedback delivered by the sense organs. A lot of adaptability is needed when a lost part of an arm is supplanted by a prosthesis. In this case it has been found (Moberg) that maintained skin sensitivity of the stump is decisive for establishing control by feedback over the mechanical instrument.[56]

The motor units of the legs in many mammals are gathered into "heads" or muscles of dominantly tonic or phasic nature. The tonic ones contract slowly and are capable of long-lasting steady efforts of limited strength; the phasic muscles are capable of handling heavier loads and of acting rapidly but are more fatigable than the tonic ones. In newborn kittens there is an incipient differentiation into two types, but both are still slowly contracting. If at that stage the nerves to two leg muscles, one phasic and the other tonic, are exchanged, what will happen? (Buller, Eccles, and Eccles)[57] Will the slow nonfatigable muscle become fast when provided with the axons of motoneurons for the fast muscle and will the fast muscle remain slow when innervated by axons destined for a slow muscle?

The experimental reply was that within considerable limits they would exchange properties. In the first instance this implies that the motoneuron exercises a decisive influence on the contractile properties of the muscle fibers on which it synapses (motor end plates). Thus, in a recent experiment, on cross-innervation of the slow soleus and the fast extensor digitorum longus muscles in the leg of the rat, it was found that reciprocal changes took place in contractile properties and in the concentration of the enzyme acting on the muscle substance myosin (Bárány and Close).[58] The myosin of the crossed extensor digitorum longus was now found to be very similar to that of the normal slow soleus, while the myosin of the crossed soleus was very similar to that of the normal fast extensor digitorum longus. There are many histochemically traceable differences between slow and fast motor units. The fast ones, for instance, make more use of glycogen, a kind of sugar broken down anaerobically by glycolytic enzymes; the slow ones are richly provided with oxidative enzymes for enduring maintenance of function. The demonstration by Romanul and Van Der Meulen that cross-innervation leads to a corresponding reversal of the histochemical profiles of slow and fast muscles has been confirmed many times.[59]

The powerful effect of a motoneuron upon the muscle fibers on which it has synapses is of the greatest interest in the present connection as a living model of how a substrate can be labeled by chemical transposition across a synapse. It illustrates a principle also available for explaining other aspects of adaptability of central neurons influenced by other neurons: the existence of "markers" conducted across synapses; though, thinking of neurons, we do not know if they merely penetrate to the synapse, or as far as the subsynaptic receptor within the cell membrane, or perhaps even into the interior of the cell.

Processes of chemical labeling conducted through nerve fibers are being hotly pursued today by the experimenters engaged in the study of axoplasmic flow.[60] Slow transport along nerve fibers of such material as neurohormones and enzymes is well established, and this process at least partly explains the transformations muscle fibers undergo in cross-innervation experiments. The other conducted event, the nerve impulse, apparently plays a role too. The influence of the nerve impulse on contractile properties stems from the rate and duration at which a discharge is emitted from the motoneuron. The impulse in motor fibers of different mammals is conducted at rates from 40 to 90 m/sec, while axoplasmic flow takes place at rates from about 1 to 240 mm a day.

Concluding Remarks

What has been said so far does not exhaust the subject of adaptability in the nervous system. Every adaptation to environmental factors can in fact be treated from the point of view of adaptability. My aim is not completeness but rather to introduce the subject of adaptability by a few examples based on developmental neurobiology. This also illustrates how testing of the phenotype works out in cases in which it has been possible to entertain some well-founded notions as to how repurposing might be achieved. They underline my basic argument that teleological purposiveness cannot be neglected in genetics if, as that science claims, the testing of mutations and recombination takes place in the phenotype.

It has been shown that the phylogenetic development of adaptability reaches its climax in parallel with the expansion of the cortex or roof brain up to its greatest size in man. Even leaving out consciousness, this whole development of adaptability is one of the most remarkable phenomena that biology is called upon to explain. The examples were chosen to indicate the nature of some biological explanations that deserve to be ranked high. The organizational explanation based on error correction by feedback places rules of repurposing in the realm of cybernetics, the science of regulation.[34] This attempt at rationalizing the problem is translatable into experiments. But general regulating principles do not absolve us from trying to understand the nature of the specific biological processes obeying the constraints of cybernetic theory. It is well known that regulated, interconnected mechanical, electrical, and biological events conform to the same general rules of cybernetics.

In looking for cellular substrates serving adaptability as well as its complement, specification, or fixation of a response, I chose to embrace Jacobson's view according to which the Golgi II cell types with short processes are "unspecified" and the Golgi I types with long axons are once and for all "specified." The former are numerous enough for their task. Methods of counting the total number of neurons in the cortex of man may not be very precise, but the range of figures from 2.6×10^9 to 14×10^9 is likely to be an estimate of the right order of magnitude. Some figures have been given for synaptic density and connectivity. The cellular mass of small neurons is not amorphous; on the contrary, it is structurally organized in conjunction with the larger cells.

The experiments on cross-innervation provide evidence for a conducted process of chemical labeling. A number of synaptic transmitter substances are known, but in addition the small cells may be chemically differentiated in the manner of the lymphocytes of the immune system. We have no information on this point. We do know, however, that intercellular separation can be modified by growth and detraction. Such phenomena are of particular importance for understanding the effects of use or disuse, which are being studied a great deal in developmental neurobiology today.[61] It seems entirely possible that in the act of repurposing a path could be expanded to reach new contacts by use while the original connection is disconnected and so "depurposed" from its original role by disuse.

Purpose, chance, and causality concern points of view rather than the actual hardware. The total causality involved in a purposive response can be subdivided into an inside complex (such as memory, genetical instructions, or fixed circuits), which only rarely will be fully known, and an external component relating the response to the environmental stimulus. Purpose or no purpose, the physics of the stimulus is the same and decisive up to the point when it is taken care of by the cellular operator, of whose resources we now have caught a glimpse. At the moment purposiveness comes closest to a role of practical usefulness in the error-detection and feedback-correction hypothesis outlined. An important consequence of this hypothesis is its requirement for communication in at least two and often more directions. But the essential secrets are well preserved by the adaptable or plastic small cells that are modifiable in connectivity by experience. Their exceedingly great number, while indicating their importance, is also a serious obstacle for the analyst. Because induced changes persist, at least as long as some environmental conditioning is being maintained, the small cells have a history and what they remember has also been influenced by unpredictable chance factors. They can never be neglected in discussing memory. But then what does memory involve, how creative is chance, and to what extent are single cells individualized? Questions of this sort could be multiplied if my intention had been to expose our ignorance rather than to present some means and ways of approaching these exciting problems.

4
Encephalization, Cortical Maps, and Redundancy

If we refuse to admit that discrimination is in some way based on different anatomical constituents differently located in the brain, we may as well give up altogether. (Author, in his Silliman Lectures, published as *Receptors and Sensory Perception*, by Yale University Press, 1955.)

Encephalization

The highly developed adaptability of man, as studied in Chapter 3, suggests that perfection of this talent could be ascribed to the existence of a roof brain or cortex greater than that of other mammals. While this structure has acquired the role of a supreme governor, it has also had to become cognizant of whatever happens outside the body or inside it (Chapter 8), which, of course, presupposes that it is informed by messages from its sense organs or in some cases by changes of blood chemistry. The role of information is to elicit action, most of it motor. For this reason Sherrington considered that the biological origin of the mind was its usefulness for motor acts.[62]

Developing in size and importance, the roof brain took over checking processes that in phylogenetically primitive vertebrates were wholly governed by lower stations. This is often spoken of as an increasing degree of encephalization (corticalization) or in some old papers as von Monakow's law of movement (that is, of controlling functions) to the higher centers. For example, the pyramidal path descending from the cortical motor area is a puny tract in the rat, but it contains about 186,000 fibers in the cat and is a mighty bundle of 1.2 million fibers in man. A more surprising example is the fact that the retina of the frog differentiates edges and direction of movement with the aid of individual ganglion cells, something that a monkey can do only with cells in its cortex (Chapter 6).

The growth of the skull from the hominids to ourselves, *Homo sapiens*, is illustrated in Figure 4.1 (Kurtén).[63] Modern methods of dating fossils have made it possible to plot size of brain cavity against geological time. The brain of the hominids (*Australopithecus*) scarcely increased at all in size

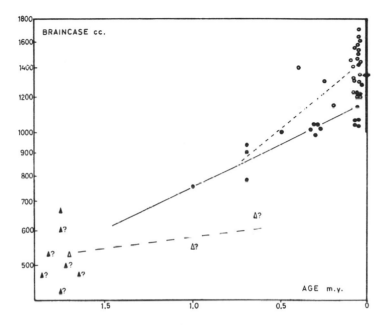

4.1. Semilogarithmic diagram representing braincase volume and absolute age in millions of years in 50 fossil hominid skulls (open triangles, *Australopithecus robustus*; filled triangles, *A. africanus*; open circles, Neanderthal group; filled circles, *Homo erectus* group). Question marks indicate doubtful age or size. Continuous line: *H. erectus* regression. Upper dashed line: regression for Neanderthal group combined with early *H. erectus* (older than 0.4 million years). Lower dashed line: approximate *Australopithecus* trend. Mean and range for modern *H. sapiens* indicated along right margin of graph. From Björn Kurtén. *Commentationes Biologicae Soc. Sci. Fenn.* (1971), 36.

before this species died out. Its growth rate is given as
about 1 to 2 percent for 100,000 years. *Homo erectus* had a
considerably faster rate of skull growth, 4.6 percent each
100,000 years. With *Homo Neanderthalensis* the rate rose to
7.5 percent each 100,000 years. The thickened ordinate on
the right, marked by cross-strokes, shows the average size
of our brain (1,350 cc) and its range of variation. If size
alone were decisive, we would in the average be worse off
by about 100 cc than the Neanderthal man. Actually, development also concerns specific sites of expansion and internal organization. The kinks in the curve suggest lack of
data or unexplained genetic revolutions. The leading view
seems to be that expansion precedes differentiation, which
then fills out the room available somewhat in the manner
of Parkinson's law: work (function) expands to fill the time
(space) available for it! Perhaps development of language
can explain the rise responsible for the Neanderthalian increase from 4.6 percent to 7.5 percent each 100,000 years.

A gradual increase in the size of the body is likely to be a
factor in the pre-Neanderthalian curve. On the average,
brain weight B is proportional to body weight W raised to
an exponent 0.63 ($B = kW^{0.63}$). Much the same relation
prevails between body weight and body surface so that the
decisive factor apparently is the surface an animal turns toward the external world. A species-dependent factor k expresses the degree of encephalization. The literature on
this subject is interesting.[64] "The encephalization of man is
higher than that of all other mammals so far investigated"
(Stephan, p. 162). There is a large gap between recent non-
human primates (higher apes) with an encephalization
factor of 10 and man with one of 30.

The increase of brain size in these terms is responsible
for the success of our highly adaptable species, though, as

pointed out by Dobzhansky, there are considerable variations from the mean (1,350 cc) that indicate a large margin of tolerance.[24] For example, of the ranges in brain volume, Jonathan Swift, 2,000 cc, and Anatole France, 1,100 cc, were cited. The late Beritoff had a remarkable case, a microcephalic girl brought to the hospital at an age of approximately 8 to 10 years, parents unknown.[65] After she died at 10 to 12, the brain was subjected to a postmortem examination. The two hemispheres weighed 289 g (normal 1,160 g); its cortical surface measured 44,041 mm as against 173,782 mm in a child of age 10 to 11. The brain stem was only 7 g below that of a child of her age. This girl did not learn to speak, nor was she capable of elementary planned behavior such as reaching for food with a cane. She reacted adequately to stimulation of all sense organs, displayed emotional manifestations, and some vocalization. Her capacity for learning corresponded roughly to that of a dog. Beritoff concluded that the number, connectivity, and organization of the cortical elements "were perfectly sufficient for psychoneural activity characteristic of higher vertebrates; they were not sufficient for eliciting the human type of planned psychoneural behaviour" (p. 53). Microcephaly is reviewed by Halloway.[66]

Because there are no fossil brains, we can compare cortical areas in man and orangutan, two land animals of much the same size with many features in common. Both have convoluted or "corrugated" (Le Gros Clark's expression) brains; that is, they possess the gyri and sulci that anatomists and physiologists use as important landmarks in brain research. Lower in the phylum this mode of cortical expansion is absent. The rabbit, for instance, has a smooth cortex; the cat a corrugated one.

If one compares those areas of Table 4.1 in ape and man

Table 4.1 Area of Regions of Cerebral Cortex

Lobes	Orangutan	Man
Occipital	47	103
Inferior parietal	9	79
Limbic	9	17
Precentral	42	63
Frontal	33	208
Temporal	100	193
Miscellaneous		177
Total	240 cm²	840 cm²

Source: D. Ploog and T. Melnechuk in *Neurosci. Res. Symp.* 6 (1970).

that are largely motor in function (the precentral ones), the difference is not large. The great expansion is reserved for the frontal, temporal, and parietal fields that represent complex functions. This line of development is seen from another angle in Figure 4.2. Although the rat and the ground shrew have cortical areas committed largely to motor action or sensory projections, the rest of the cortex (white in the figure) increases from monkey to man. Speech, for instance, concerns the temporal and inferior parietal lobes, which are much larger in man than in the orangutan. Extensive areas are devoted to "higher functions," as I will show.

Maps and Mapping

The idea of a cortical localization of specific functions had to fight its way to recognition against the notion prevailing at the end of the last century that the cortex was functionally uniform.[67] Most serious disputes in science, like this one,

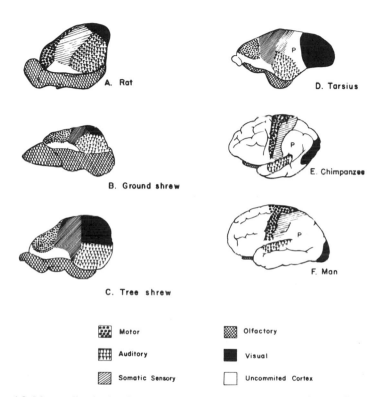

A. Rat

B. Ground shrew

C. Tree shrew

D. Tarsius

E. Chimpanzee

F. Man

▨ Motor   ▨ Olfactory

▦ Auditory   ■ Visual

▨ Somatic Sensory   ☐ Uncommited Cortex

4.2. Mammalian brains from rat to man prepared by Stanley Cobb to illustrate the proportional increase of uncommitted cortex (or undetermined cortex) as compared with sensory and motor cerebral cortex.

do not end in absolute victory for one side. In this case our thinking has acquired nuances from new techniques based on electronics, the science responsible for the use of both microelectrodes and the electron microscope. We now realize that there are highly localized functions, even tricks—if I may say so—that only certain aggregates of cells can perform, as well as functions that require a coactivation of several widely separated cortical areas. Delving into problems of localization, we tend to end up with problems of organization. In a general way one may say that the more complex the function defined, the more neural space it seems to occupy in all dimensions.

The "wiring" of the sensory projections to the cortex has been studied in detail by electrical methods of stimulation and recording, and maps of the primary end stations have been published, two of which are shown in Figures 4.3 and 4.4. The large somatic sensory area (Figure 4.4) whose anterior portion overlaps with the motor area (both shown in Figure 4.3) provides us with the basic geographic knowledge of our body surface. The visual area (Figure 4.4) similarly represents the external world projected on the retinal surface, the binocular overlapping part as well as the smaller monocular portions; the somatic sensory area reproduces the body surface.

Such primary sensory projections do not represent sites of conscious perception. Rather, they should be called sites of sensation to distinguish these areas from those required for full perceptual elaboration aided by memory. The primary areas are chiefly to be regarded as junctions on the route in which some reorganization of incoming messages takes place. Stimulating them electrically in man does not lead to perception of anything meaningful. From the visual area there are reports of "flickering lights, dancing lights,

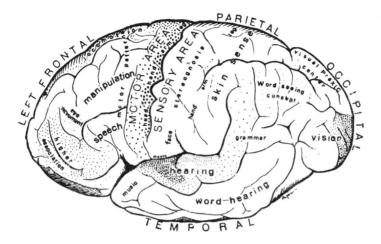

4.3. Lateral view of the left cerebral hemisphere showing functional localization. From James W. Papez, *Comparative Neurology* (New York: Crowell, 1929).

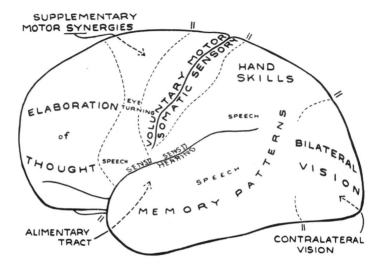

4.4. Representation, according to a Congress Report by the late Wilder Penfield, of the localization of certain functions in the dominant hemisphere of man.

colors, bright lights, stars, wheels, blue, green and red colored discs, fawn and blue lights, colored bells whirling, radiating grey spots becoming pink and blue, a long white mark et cetera" (Penfield and Rasmussen, p. 145).[67] The same authors mention reports of sensations from patients whose somatic sensory area has been stimulated: "tingling, electricity, numbness, sense of movement" referred to specific parts on the opposite side of the body (pathways being crossed). Complete meaningful sequences of perceptions elicited by electrical stimulation were obtained merely from the temporal lobe. Thus what Penfield and Rasmussen found in the primary projections were fragments of an organization that since has been studied in considerable detail by microelectrodes (see Chapters 6 and 9).

Localization in the areas of elaboration, often called "association areas" (Figure 4.3) cannot be defined with the same amount of precision. The terms in which they are described in the figures refer to mental operations that acquire full meaning only with human subjects, but then of course we are interested in ourselves, and these areas are also much larger in man than in other animals. They do not respond to electrical stimulation in the manner of primary projection areas. Sensory and motor elaboration is needed, for instance, for skillful hand movements and for speech, but electrical stimulation of those areas merely stops performance. The temporal cortex with its peculiar access to things remembered is an exception (Chapter 5). For this reason much of what is known about elaboration areas has come from patients with head injuries, epilepsy, or ablations in conjunction with testing procedures, for example, and consequently is somewhat anecdotal. Clearly these areas are activated from the inside. Much of our information about them cannot be reviewed without knowledge of anatomy and physiology beyond the level of presentation in this book. Recent attempts at analyzing cellular responses in these areas will be taken up in Chapter 9. Though the huge expansion of the cortex distinguishes man from other species in the phylum, we share with other mammals the subcortical structures, just as we also share with them states of sleep and wakefulness, emotional attitudes, and basic reflexes of orientation and posture. As we shall see, subcortical components participate in all our responses to the environment and sometimes acquire a dominant role (discussed separately in Chapters 9 and 10). In preparing a background for some general comments on the principles of localization we are, however, best served by presenting the necessary facts in terms of results from the field of cortical physiology.[68]

General Significance of Cell Number

Importance, precision, and detailed specification are aspects of localization that within any particular cortical area are furthered by an augmentation of the number of participating cells. This is shown in brief outline by the homunculi of the motor and sensory fields of Figures 4.5 and 4.6. The large face and hand areas of the sensory and motor fields represent the need for highly discriminative sensitivity and finely controlled motor action respectively. The representation of the fovea of the eye demonstrates the same principle for the visual area, for which some figures are available.

In monkeys, in the foveal part of the retina, which is its most important focusing region, 2 minutes of visual angle at the retina is rerepresented within a millimeter at the cortex, whereas at 5° toward the periphery of vision as much as 18 minutes of visual angle are squeezed into the same width of 1 mm cortical projection. A circle of 1 minute visual angle encloses 0.005 mm at the fovea. It is multiplied 10,000 times at the cortex where it corresponds to a circle of 0.5 mm.[69] Thus the region of optimal vision in daylight is analyzed at the cortex by magnification based on multiplying cell numbers. And this is merely one of the first brain sites where some reorganization of the sensory message takes place before it is delivered to other portions of the brain for an elaboration I call perception. Small wonder that the brain needs millions and millions of cells if this is how it is organized for high-grade performance. Functional studies of the visual area will be dealt with in Chapter 6, but for the moment let us remain within anatomy.

There are about 2 million fibers in the two optic nerves of man, some 38 percent of our total sensory input. Reorganized for binocular vision, these project on to the lateral geniculate body, an intermediate station in the thalamus in the midst of the brain. Any single fiber from the geniculate body has terminals on 5,000 neurons in the primary visual area, and each of these neurons is in contact with 4,000 other neurons (Sholl).[49] Thus there is interaction, and interaction is the raison d'être of cellular multiplication. For the individual cells interaction may be in the nature of an enhancement (excitation) or a suppression (inhibition) of their activity. The nature of such interactions can in specific cases be analyzed by electrical techniques, as has been done for primary visual projection (Chapter 6) and the motor area (Chapter 8). At this point the problem of localization turns into an analysis of organization that should indicate what precisely is the function that is being localized.

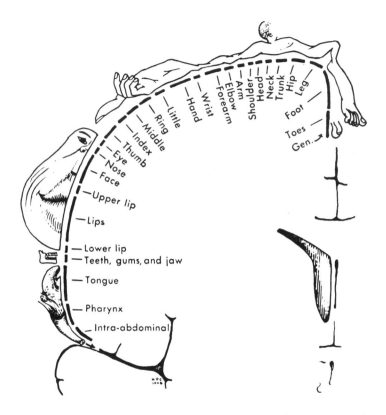

4.5. Sensory homunculus. The right side of the figure is on a cross-section of the hemisphere, drawn somewhat in proportion to the extent of sensory cortex devoted to it. The length of the underlying block lines indicates more accurately the comparative extent of each representation. Compare with 4.6. From Wilder Penfield and Theodore Rasmussen, *The Cerebral Cortex of Man* (New York: Macmillan, 1950).

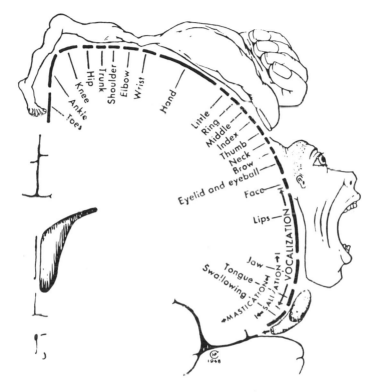

4.6. Motor homunculus. The right side of the figure is on a cross-section of the hemisphere. Compare with 4.5. From Wilder Penfield and Theodore Rasmussen, *The Cerebral Cortex of Man* (New York: Macmillan, 1950).

Redundancy

Like negative feedback, redundancy emphasizes an aspect of cellular multiplication that belongs to general principles rather than to any particular locus in the central nervous system. It means that a central response, indeed, even that of a single cell in the visual cortex, is supported by a greater number of pathways and neurons than it actually needs to function. Redundancy is a concept that biology shares with communication engineering.* In his less formalized and more empirical approach the physiologist also realizes that Nature takes no chances with anything important. Everywhere one finds important functions secured by a redundancy of pathways and also by a multiplicity of mechanisms capable of producing much the same end effect. The engineer who is a reasonably good imitator of Nature's tricks also uses redundancy, but on a considerably smaller scale. For example, though "individual wires going to each telephone are necessary for function . . . deep inside the exchange there are many 'senders' any of which can assume various functions. If only a few of them are disconnected, there would be little or no noticeable functional difference in the exchange. It would be a little bit slow in answering or setting up some of the calls, but these behavioral deficits would be detectable only through very subtle tests" (Shannon).[70] Similarly, as sometimes happens when the neurosurgeon has been forced to remove the cerebellum, a large

---

*In information theory the amount of information or "entropy" is defined by the letter H in Shannon's formula (see any textbook in the field, e.g., F. H. George, *Cybernetics and Biology*. Edinburgh and London: Oliver & Boyd, 1965). Redundancy is the complement of information that could have been passed relative to the amount that actually was communicated. With the aid of the formula it can be measured quantitatively.

organ with some 10 billion cells, very special tests may be required to detect an abnormality of gait if the patient is allowed to keep his eyes open and thus has access to visual compensatory control. The electronic engineer is much concerned about the irregular low-level activity in his circuits called "noise" because his signal must exceed the noise level. There is much spontaneous activity going on in the afferent input to the central nervous system; this has also been regarded as biological noise. In the nervous system, as in other circuits, a message has to exceed the noise level. Redundancy is one organizational feature by which noise is counteracted but there are others, particularly mechanisms based on inhibition, which is of fundamental importance at several levels as a filter enhancing the relevance of a message by restructuring it.

The central nervous system by no means behaves as a passive receiver of input (Chapter 9). It selects its information actively by processing it in the periphery, at the subcortical level, and within the cortex, where the ultimate selection takes place with the aid of consciousness. The mechanisms for rejection of noise are so highly developed that the physiological problem bears a merely superficial likeness to that of the communication engineer. Spontaneous impulse activity plays a most important role by maintaining a certain level of facilitation in the cells. Against this background of increased excitability nervous inhibition has a chance of modulating a response for greater pregnancy with regard to the permanently or momentarily needful. As yet no mathematics are available to formalize the role of cell multiplication in localizing highly discriminative responses because the fundamental variables of a quantitative treatment would have to be known. We are still too

ignorant about them to use the mathematical instrument.
To make some preliminary sense out of these intricate organizations, the investigator has to rely on an empirical
approach with the aid of electrical recording and on behavioral abnormalities in man or animals with verifiable local
destructions.

Expansion, Encephalization, and Localization

The three general aspects of cortical physiology surveyed
clearly have a purpose in common that is best illustrated by
referring to the localization of the structures handling
speaking and the understanding of language (marked
speech in Figure 4.4). The language areas have long been
known to be located in the left hemisphere, but the two
hemispheres are also connected by a system of communicating fibers, the corpus callosum, which permits them to
cooperate harmoniously (see Chapter 5). Whether this
communication with the right hemisphere meant anything
for the understanding of language was until fairly recently
unknown. There are pathological cases in which surgical
section of the corpus callosum has been a justifiable cure;
in them it has been possible to demonstrate that the right
hemisphere actually is incapable of communicating by language while its left partner remains in full possession of
this talent (next chapter and note 81). It is thus possible to
compare the anatomy of corresponding regions, one with
and the other without a role in communication. The two
sites in the left and the right hemisphere are actually highly
asymmetrical, the left side containing the speech areas, being both larger and more richly differentiated (Geschwind).[53] In a small number of people speech is represented in both hemispheres. What this implies in the way of

anatomical development is at the moment unknown.
The question of what is being localized—which will concern us in specific cases in the next chapters—has been pursued along two main lines: (1) the neurophysiological, tightly stimulus-bound, experimental approach, and (2) the other proceeding to some kind of understanding by psychological definitions (in man) or using behavioral observations (in animals) in the belief that the recorded motor reactions would not as such contribute essentially to the behavioral act. While we are aiming at combining—as far as it goes—neurophysiological and anatomical knowledge with clinical experience and psychological or behavioral responses, there is a limit beyond which only psychology can take over, aided in some cases by anatomy, and possibly caught up in a distant future by neurophysiology. An example of this is speech, as spoken and understood. At their best the neurophysiological analyses of today carry us to the level of the primary projections in the visual, acoustic, somatic, and other sensory areas and sometimes a bit beyond them.

Our present knowledge of localized functions in the brain is steadily expanding. Modern anatomy is at a high technical level. It makes use of refined staining methods aided by improved light microscopy and the electron microscope. In the last instance, however, a functional criterion is needed to define what is being localized. At the moment we are trying to understand encoding and decoding of information, mechanisms of cellular interaction, what fraction of experience is handled by a single cell, how conscious percepts result from available bits of information, and a host of other questions.

In relation to the enormous task of understanding nervous action and perception, the insight laid down in the principle of differentiation by localization may seem insignificant as an attempt at classifying brain activity. Nevertheless it serves as the backbone on which the rest of our body of knowledge hinges.

Another matter is then how to proceed to the next step in classification and decide to what class of phenomena a living nervous system belongs. It is a unique phenomenon in this world—unique also in ultimately trying to understand itself.

5
Some Approaches to
Conscious Awareness

Any science that deals with living organisms must needs cover the phenomenon of consciousness, because consciousness, too, is part of reality. (Niels Bohr in a discussion recorded by Heisenberg in *Physics and Beyond*, London: Allen and Unwin, 1971, p. 114.)

The introductory quotation illustrates the agreement of two physicists of the first rank (Bohr and Heisenberg) on what many of those with some experience of neurophysiology regard as self-evident. Others think of consciousness as an epiphenomenon or as something that merely has semantic existence. I do not intend to spend any arguments on them. From the evolutionary standpoint of modern biology, consciousness is an emergent novelty, probably still existing in an increasingly rudimentary form as one descends in the phylum. Sherrington, speaking of mind and often meaning consciousness, regarded it as a product of evolution, developing from unrecognizable to recognizable with no lower limit accessible to definition.[62] He held mind to have arisen in connection with the motor act whose improvement gave it survival value. A similar attitude based on evolution is that of Teilhard de Chardin (1955) who cut the Gordian knot by simply maintaining that "toute énergie est de nature psychique."[71] However, a more tangible approach than this is needed.

A better differentiated version of the evolutionary attitude is that of Polanyi who, in agreement with Hughlings Jackson,[4] Paul Weiss,[3] the present author, and many others, emphasizes creation of hierarchies as a component of evolutionary progress: "the principles governing the isolated particulars of a lower level leave indeterminate conditions to be controlled by a higher principle. Voice production leaves largely open the combination of sounds into words, which is controlled by a vocabulary. Next, a vocabulary leaves largely open the combination of words to form sentences, which is controlled by grammar, and so on. Consequently, the operations of a higher level cannot be accounted for by the laws governing its particulars on the next lower level. You cannot derive a vocabulary from phonetics; you cannot derive grammar from a vocabulary; a correct use of grammar does not account for good style; and a good style does not supply the content of a piece of prose" (p. 1311).[72] This analogy shows how conscious man makes use of neurophysiological mechanisms without being governed by them.[73] In an analogous way a computer makes use of the laws governing electrical circuits, so-called hardware, but the purpose embodied in its design cannot be reduced to terms of hardware without losing its relevance.

Neverthcless we have to know the principles utilized by Nature in the choice of hardware, as well as the hardware itself down to the last limit of reductionism, because all these facts and rules of operation impose constraints on the phenomenon of conscious awareness without directly being awareness as such. When, for instance, we observe that consciousness is lost in deep sleep, the conclusion that it is tied to cellular processes subject to inhibition can be justified, but this does not define its nature; it merely fixes one particular constraint. In the same way Sherrington's statement that consciousness seems to develop in parallel with the expansion of the cerebral cortex—a likely hypothesis— defines another boundary condition. Such facts are often interesting and important in themselves as contributions to physiology and its application in medicine, but they do not explain the phenomenon of conscious awareness. And how could they? To deliver a conscious explanation of the essence of consciousness involves a feat such as Baron von Münchausen's lifting himself and his horse out of a morass by his own queue. "We cannot reach further than to understand what can be understood and realize what we cannot understand" (Berzelius, introductory quotation to Chapter 1). Often the unavoidability of a concept or attitude is more important even than full understanding of all its implications. When I consciously demand from myself the performance of a complex motor act, "demand" is a useful concept embodying certain constraints; but in spite of this I may not understand what "demanding" is. To this general category belongs "conscious awareness," whereas "mind" epitomizes a general desire to deal with experience from one particular point of view. It means that we intend to classify our material in psychological terms. We then keep to the hierarchic top level of organization, the evolutionary summit that serves as a carrier of the whole of our civilization taken in the widest possible sense of that word.

Evolutionary Assets of Consciousness

As held already by William James, conscious awareness is a process engaged in evaluating the resources of a brain that has grown too complex to do itself justice without it.[74] In this respect, what other advantages could it tender a neural machinery that does so well without it?*

1. Consciousness makes possible long-range anticipation of events. Anticipation is tied to purposive acts in which, as we shall see, it also may become automatic. However, my emphasis here is on the great expansion in two dimensions, time and complexity of association, that consciousness alone can engender. Because no anticipation is possible

---

*"The *distribution* of consciousness shows it to be exactly such as we might expect in an organ added for the sake of steering a nervous system grown too complex to regulate itself." (James, p. 144.)

without predictability, perhaps one of the most remarkable properties of consciousness is that it has supplied a high degree of predictability to an organism that in ontogeny has undergone the hardships of genetic chance, environmental challenges, and developmental interactions between its parts.

2. Time runs through the whole world of biology, but consciousness has added an element of awareness to it. A dog can be trained to use a time interval as a stimulus in conditioned reflexes but, over and above that, man has introduced the notion of the past and the future to characterize experience.

3. Consciousness can raise to the level of awareness most sensory experiences and an incredible number of engrams (memories). It therefore serves as an activator capable of selecting cells and circuits and keeping them in focus to the exclusion of others. This again means that it makes use of both excitation and inhibition.

4. Given time, consciousness can deal with vast amounts of information. No animal can compete with man though higher mammals may be equal to man in pure associative learning.

5. However, learning complex matters presupposes conscious awareness which therefore plays a definite role in stamping in engrams.

6. Consciousness is necessary for the development of communication at the level of man.

7. Consciousness facilitates correction of misinterpretations or errors including those of automatized acts.

8. As pointed out in discussing adaptability, consciousness reigns supreme in this regard. In adaptability conscious man exceeds all other species.

Conscious awareness has been an enormous asset in the

evolution of higher organisms. Its raison d'être is perfection of control over the environment—and indeed, some today believe that in man it has become too successful.

Timing Consciousness

Patients in whom the sensorimotor area of the cortex has been partially laid bare for surgical purposes have allowed the surgeon to stimulate it electrically. The electrodes have been applied to the bared surface or pushed slightly into the white matter of nerve fibers below it. The procedure is painless. In such experiments by Libet and his colleagues it turned out that although each shock elicited a virtually instantaneous electrical cell response, an evoked potential, it required a whole series of shocks before the patient registered conscious awareness of the stimulus in the form of a percept.[75] In fact, the interval or latent period was as long as half a second. Because the cortical cells were activated instantaneously they could hardly have been the sole neuronal substrate of the much-delayed conscious response. This agrees with the experience of neurosurgeons. Therefore, as Penfield points out, any portion of the cerebral cortex can be removed without causing loss of consciousness. It is, however, inevitably lost when the function of the higher portion of the brain stem is interrupted by injury, pressure, disease, or local epileptic discharge.

The latent period of the conscious response suggests that coengagement of the brain stem by a network of nervous loops is the most elementary assumption one can make to explain the onset and disappearance of awareness of an event that one has good reasons for localizing to the cortical gray matter. It also means that when afferent nerve stimuli elicit fast movements, they are well underway before one becomes aware of them. This is true not only of reflexes but of acquired skillful responses as well. Such movements can now be traced at several sites by electrical recording within the brain, spinal cord, and muscles of monkeys. Formerly the experimenters were restricted to measuring the reaction time of human subjects, which implicitly was regarded as a conscious response indicated by the motor act of pressing a Morse key. Now it seems likely that this act, too, is completed long before it has reached the level of conscious awareness. Reaction times are of the order of 0.1 to 0.2 sec. If Libet and his coworkers are right about awareness requiring about half a second, then conscious recording of the act of pressing a key must succeed the motor response and turn up after the completion of the reaction time. In favor of this conclusion is the observation of psychologists (Craik; Vince)[76] that the least interval between the conscious identification of two visual stimuli as doubles is of the order of half a second, a figure in good agreement with a latent period of the same order, as Libet's group found.

It will be shown with examples in subsequent chapters that whenever motor acts or perceptions have been properly analyzed, they have been found to involve a very large number of neurons in different parts of the brain. For this reason and because of the involvement of the brainstem, it also seems likely that conscious awareness as a process necessarily implicates a vast number of cells from different sites. The long latent period would be largely caused by the mobilization of this elaborate cellular apparatus. Physiologists call the act of mobilizing the brain "arousal." They record its electrical signs and hold arousal to be an important neural component in stirring up attention that is excited by the appearance of some object of interest. The trend of evolution seems to have favored the capacity of making conscious use of attention. We feel it in our power to direct our attention to anything we choose to consider.[77]

Signs of Conscious Mentation and of Arousal

When speaking of signs in this sense, I mean events that can be measured and even produced in various ways by the objective method of psychophysiology. Generally known is the electroencephalogram (Berger) obtainable by recording with electrodes placed on the scalp.[78] This has the character of synchronized waves of potential changes across membranes of neurons including their dendritic expansions. In the state of rest there is a basic rhythm, 10 per second, on which are superposed irregular wavelets. One of Berger's early observations was that these waves grow smaller and reach higher frequencies when the subject's attention is engaged. The state of deep sleep is characterized by slow waves of large size, the electroencephalogram of the active awake subject by smaller and faster waves. These changes are seen also in animals and are similarly interpreted as signs of sleep and awareness, with the additional requirement that behavioral signs of awareness must also be present to indicate that the animal really has been alerted.

A descriptive science of electrophenomenology has been erected on the basis of electroencephalography. This has become useful in the clinic for localizing tumors and epileptic tendencies and states, but beyond underlining our conviction that conscious awareness is tied to cellular activity it does not tell us anything about its nature. The dead brain is electrically silent. The living brain responds with electrical signs of alertness (arousal) to electrical stimulation of the brainstem within a region whose role seems to be to collect branches from all incoming (afferent) fibers from the various sense organs and to make use of the information obtained through them to activate the cortex of the entire cerebrum (Magoun's reticular activating system.)[77] In the absence of this system, permanent sleep ensues.

The electroencephalographic technique of recording brain waves by electrodes on the skull of man has recently been much improved by using computers for electronic summation of otherwise invisible changes of potential. A sensory stimulus, for instance a visual contrast pattern, would produce a minute change of potential but this alteration would be lost in the noise consisting of the background wavelets of the living brain. However, by repeating the stimulus, say, up to 200 times, the computer would sum the minute changes of each test until its effect has become recordable. Some results of such work will be mentioned in the next two chapters. Its main interest in the present connection is that the method has revealed long-lasting electrical changes during mentation, such as in the state of expectancy or waiting for something to happen (Grey Walter).[79] (See Chapter 9.) In connection with different psychologically defined operations the method is of interest for problems concerning timing, duration, and elementary localization of otherwise inaccessible processes. It can be used also to measure the intensity or degree of a process and is thus a valuable asset for the science of psychophysiology. On the whole it seems likely that this branch of physiology faces a time of expansion.

Engrams, Communication, and Levels of Awareness

Much could be added on the role of consciousness in different connections but I shall restrict myself to some interesting cases. One is Penfield's observation that large strips of awareness of long-since forgotten incidents can be revived in conscious patients by electrical stimulation of the temporal region of the bared cortex, made accessible for surgical purposes.[80] To what place the effect of the stimulus is conducted is not known, but the effect is in the nature of a remembered awareness of an experience that is reincarnated as such, despite the patient's parallel awareness of being on the surgeon's table in a hospital. The remembered incident may be complete, as it evolved in time many years earlier, and it possesses its original emotional tone, as if it had been stored in a sequence and been sealed off as originally experienced. Somehow the electrical stimulus must have facilitated access to it. In daily life we often speak of remembering in the sense of becoming conscious of something deposited in the past, but as such memory is a much wider concept.

A still more interesting case concerns observations by Sperry and his coworkers on the split brain.[81] This operation separates the outwardly symmetrical halves of the brain. It involves sectioning the main bridge between them (corpus callosum) whose 200 million nerve fibers pass information making it possible for the two hemispheres to function as one single brain. This surgical incision was carried out in certain epileptics for whom it has been of great curative value. By taking proper precautions the two hemispheres can in these patients be stimulated independently using separate eyes. What is led to the left half-brain reaches the speech center, which in virtually all people is in that hemisphere. The right half-brain is mute in the sense that its communication by language with the experimenter is undeveloped. The right hemisphere perceives and comprehends something but cannot express itself verbally. But upon reading simple words, representing objects simultaneously flashed into it, it can pick them out with the hand at its disposal (the left one, because the motor paths cross). With the dominant left hemisphere controlling the right hand, there is full normal communication. Recent methods of temporally silencing either hemisphere, for example, by localized anesthesia, and investigations on people with a removed diseased hemisphere have shown the minor or mute hemisphere to possess important talents of its own.[82] It has, for instance, considerable manual dexterity in visual-spatial manipulation. An isolated right hemisphere has been found by Luria to retain musicality, to the extent of being able to compose music.

What about consciousness in such experiments? The dominant left hemisphere in possession of full powers of communication is obviously normally conscious in the sense we think of consciousness. The question in this connection is whether the mute brain with deficient communication is less conscious than its partner. Sperry and his coworkers assign to the right hemisphere a conscious awareness different from the verbalized type: "For example, while the patient was dressing and trying to pull on his trousers, the left hand (mute hemisphere) might start to work against the right (talking hemisphere) to pull the trousers down on that side. Or, the left hand, after just helping to tie the belt of the patient's robe, might go ahead on its own to untie the completed knot, whereupon the right hand would have to supervene again to retie it. The patient and his wife used to refer to the 'sinister left hand' that sometimes tried to push the wife away aggressively at the same time that the hemisphere of the right hand was trying to get her to come and help him with something." [75] With some right, Bogen (1969) states that in this problem we have barely scraped the surface of "a vast unknown." [82]

It seems probable that communication with others or internal monologizing represent high degrees of conscious awareness. Thus consciousness is not one particular state only but something that, like other nervous states and acts, runs through a scale of intensities or levels. It would not be surprising if normal levels of consciousness in a population were determined by a Gaussian distribution curve. Some people seem to maintain a much higher level of conscious awareness than others. However, we have not yet the methods for testing my hypothesis. On the other hand, we are familiar with deviations from the assumed normal degree of consciousness other than deep sleep. There is, for instance, the so-called paradoxical sleep (REM sleep, parasleep) in which the brain exhibits electrical activity reminiscent of that in wakefulness (Dement, Jouvet). [83] The experimental evidence suggests that during this state, which is perfectly normal, the subject is dreaming and thus is apparently conscious in some way. Among other things this state involves inhibition of his spinal reflexes (Pompeiano). [83] And all of us know from personal experience states between half-sleep and full awareness.

The pathology of sleep also demonstrates different levels of conscious awareness such as somnambulism (sleepwalking) and somnolism (hypnotic sleep). Henry Head points out that "a sufferer from minor epilepsy may become completely unconscious and yet remain ignorant that he has had an attack; the stream of mental processes seems to him as unbroken as that of the astonished spectators.

But during this period of unconsciousness he can carry out the most elaborate acts, guided by what appear to be reasonable though extraordinary motives."[84]

The boundaries between conscious acts and automatisms are fleeting. We see this best in practicing complex motor acts when our main endeavor is to automatize them as soon as possible. In the end consciousness is used merely as a trigger to deliver a command and, sometimes, also to select the channel for its execution. If anything goes wrong in the accomplishment of the intent, then again consciousness is mobilized to correct for the unwanted deviation.

These are some examples of the ways in which it has been possible to approach conscious awareness from the physiological end. The neuronal changes underlying consciousness are still a secret. Only some boundary conditions such as those described are known. Biochemists may like to imagine that conscious awareness depends on the release of a quite specific substance at or within a large number of neurons; molecular biologists may want to implicate nucleotides; and neurophysiologists hypothesize the existence of special neurons interspersed among the cortical cells and requiring activation from the brain stem. However, all such notions are conjectural. It only seems certain that some kind of circuitry must be postulated, as shown by the inhibitory processes at work in sleep and by the involvement of the brain stem in cortical processes (Moruzzi).[85]

The brain as a whole, and with it conscious awareness, depends on a normal inflow of sensory messages. This seems almost a corollary of the fact, mentioned in Chapter 3, that the brain contains cells whose functions are fabricated or modified by experience. Sensory deprivation, achieved by asking volunteers to dwell for some time in the dark in a soundproof room (Hebb), has a disastrous effect on normal, balanced control of the environment, implicating also conscious acts and thoughts.[86] It is likely that the enormous, cumulative transfer of knowledge from generation to generation has had and will continue to have an influence on conscious awareness. Tinbergen has reminded us of the fact that a nongenetic transfer of this kind is without precedent in biology.[87] In this respect we are Nature's guinea pigs.

The Epistemological Point of View

In presenting some physiological approaches to conscious awareness, I have avoided the ageless controversy concerning matter and mind. This does not belong to the realm of science but to that of philosophy. Descartes (1596–1650), at the dawn of modern science, formulated the dualistic version of this relationship by his assumption of two worlds "absolument distinctes," that of "esprit" (soul, spirit) which expresses itself in thought, and that of "corps" (body) characterized by "étendue" (extensiveness).[26] In this manner he lent his great authority to the perpetuation of Jean Fernel's (1497–1558) difficulty of how to account for the entry of the spirit into the body. [88] Fernel, a physician who coined the word "physiology" and advocated a scientific study of disease based on observation, solved the problem by stating that the spirit entered the body on the fortieth day after conception!

In the beginning of this century Ernst Mach, in his important *Analyse der Empfindungen*, removed the problem of matter and mind from the domain of science.[89] He stated that science is "concerned with different basic variables and different relations. This is the main issue. Neither the facts nor the functional relationships will be changed if we treat everything as conscious experience (*Bewusstseinsinhalt*) or as partly or wholly physical. The biological task of science is to provide the rational human being with as complete an orientation as possible. A different scientific ideal is nonrealistic and is also meaningless" (my translation, pp. 29–30). In essence Mach's standpoint still seems valid to me, but from the background of evolutionism and the acceptance of hierarchic order in biology in these essays it needs some amendments. Hierarchic organization implies that at each level new functional relationships are created which use lower organizational levels, as in the example given of the tongue ultimately being used in speech (Chapter 1). But the tongue cannot run the speech.

A warp of creative purposiveness is woven into the fabric of biological hierarchies with consciousness at its top level. It is one of our tasks to trace it. The scientific explanations we are pursuing should, indeed, provide what Mach called "as complete an orientation as possible." But there must be a reorientation of purpose from level to level, extreme "reductionist" molecular details at one end, physiology in its mechanistic and integrative aspects in the middle, and rules for behavior and an independent science of psychology at the other end. Many of these explanations do not and never will end in the differential equations that the physicist uses for his world of interpretation. Life creates novelty from one level to the next. We often see the same principles applied over and over again, the way the architect uses the same bricks for new ends. As scientists we are delighted when we recognize such "bricks," of which I have given some examples, but explaining means understanding the use to which they have been put in hierarchic organizations.

Science does not require dualism. "Pluralism" would be a

better word for summarizing the many-faceted aims of biological science, not in the least in its interpretations of the central nervous system. In science we do not reach out for the soul of man that "catches the gleam of sunlight as it falls on the foliage. It nurtures poetry. Men are the children of the Universe, with foolish enterprises and irrational hopes. A tree sticks to its business of mere survival; and so does an oyster with some minor divergencies. In this way, the life-aim at survival is modified into the human aim at survival for diversified worth-while experiences" (Whitehead, pp. 42–43).[90] As human beings, we may need the dualism of body and mind, matter and soul, or we may regard it as a practical way of describing experience. It is not, however, the scientific way.

6
In Search of Building Blocks
for Perception

The early unitary analysis, by H. K. Hartline[38] and the present author, of optic nerve discharges drew attention to movement-sensitivity of the retina and suggested that "[S.C. impulse] frequency must be of particular importance for the discrimination of stimulus intensity pattern, not only for this task but for the recognition of spatial phenomena such as the dominance of contour and 'local sign'. . . . The accurate appreciation of contour, in particular, must be due to minute fluctuations of the eyeballs resulting in on- and off-effects as well as sudden inhibitions of the latter. Even if it were possible to keep the eye absolutely still, every sharp intensity gradient must give rise to very complicated excitation inhibition patterns tending to emphasize the gradients and giving the higher centres a cue for discrimination." (Author in *Sensory Mechanisms of the Retina*, Oxford University Press, 1947, pp. 168–169.)

From Classical to Modern Psychophysics

The old psychophysics founded in the last century and formalized in Fechner's *Elemente der Psychophysik* (1862) is less respected today than it deserves to be.[91] What it did was to create a science out of nothingness, basing it on the idea that such impressions as light, sound, or pressure could be measured by physical equivalents representing different forms of energy. Psychological entities were thus to be linked to physically definable quantities. The fundamental units of psychophysics became those of the cgs (centimeter-gram-second) system. As any science must be judged by what it can classify, generalize, and explain, so also must classical psychophysics be defended by what it meant for subsequent developments in these respects.

To psychophysics we owe the concept of the absolute threshold of a sensation in cgs units, the minimum amount of energy needed for experiencing a sensation of light, sound, touch, or temperature. It also showed that sensations from the skin did not arise everywhere, but from specific sites unevenly distributed and in some cases referable to nerve endings. We still make regular use of the general concept of sensitivity, which is the inverse value of the absolute threshold or of any other constant criterion response. Although these definitions did not carry the new science deep into psychology, they proved useful when in the twenties development of electronics rendered possible a physicochemical approach to the study of energy transfer from input (physical) to nervous message. A stimulus-response approach was the obvious experimental answer to elementary questions regarding the nature of the process converting external energy to information. For a number of sensory end organs we have these answers today.

The definition of the difference threshold also became quite valuable. This is the amount of energy that has to be added to perceive a difference when increasing stimulus strength intensifies the background sensation against which it is measured. This problem was first recognized by E. H. Weber (1834) who added weights to increasingly larger weights and found the difference threshold always to be a constant of the order of 1 percent.[92] Translated for the visual sphere, which I shall use for presenting modern approaches to the interpretation of information from sense organs, Weber's rule means that for any brightness caused by light intensity I (energy) the difference threshold measured as ΔI obeys the relation $\Delta I/I = a$ constant. Fechner integrated this equation and ended up with the statement that a sensory function defined as perceived intensity S was proportional to the logarithm of the physical stimulus intensity I.

These ideas and conclusions are of more than historical interest because they initiated a way of thinking of stimulus quantities as encoded by different sense organs. For this reason they encouraged people to devise means of dealing with such problems. Again, when electronics in the hands of Adrian (1926) rendered objective recording of individual sensory impulses feasible, effects of stimulus strength could be measured in terms of impulse frequencies and so the logarithmic relation, derived by Fechner, could be tested.[93] In this manner the study of effects of stimulus strength carried research a little bit deeper into the "psycho" component of psychophysics, but, obviously, when complex sensory instruments like the eye and the ear are considered, scaling of intensities comprises but a fraction of what can be analyzed by objective and subjective methods joining forces. The greatest results of classical psychophysics were achieved in the study of the eye and the ear.[94] These results were inspired by the fact that the external world as seen or heard offered a richer variety of experience than, say, touch or smell. We are extremely visual animals and quite good acoustically, too, although inferior to the whale and the dolphin which have an acoustic frequency register spanning from 150 Hz to 150,000 Hz, whereas our range of 20 to 18,000 Hz. Compared with us, these intelligent animals have enormous acoustic projections in their brains and use high-frequency echo-sounding (radar) for communication and long-distance orientation.

The psychophysics of vision based its knowledge firmly on the wavelength of energy distribution of the perceived spectrum: red, orange, yellow, green, blue, and violet, of which the split-up white light had to be the sum. By paying attention to brightness (luminosity) alone, disregarding color, it became possible to plot a spectral distribution curve of the luminosity that overlays the chromaticity represented by specific wavelengths. This was, as it were, real psychophysics, combining a firm physical basis (wavelength and energy) with defined psychological percepts. The psychophysical science was precise enough to support a useful structure of trichromatic color-matching founded on simple algebraic laws of color mixture.

Contact was then taken up with histology which, owing to improved microscopes, rose to great prominence toward the end of the last century. The rod and cone receptors had been described in the retina. By psychophysical methods such properties as color blindness and high sensitivity in the dark were assigned to rods and color sensitivity, good visual acuity, and daylight vision to cones. This work was aided by the discovery that the fovea in the center of the human eye was rod-free and that the number of cones decreased toward the periphery of the retina. The course of adaptation to light and darkness was described with the aid of the threshold method for determining sensitivity. Soon it was also realized that the spectral luminosity (brightness) distribution was different for daylight and night vision, being in the bluish-green range for rod vision, shifting toward greenish-yellow in cone vision. Because the fovea was nightblind, it was concluded that only rods could adapt to darkness over a great range. The process of dark adaptation is virtually completed within half an hour. At about the turn of the century the photosensitive substance visual purple, today called "rhodopsin," was discovered, and its basic agreement in spectral sensitivity with the distribution of luminosity of the dark-adapted eye was confirmed. The spectral luminosity distribution of the fovea was found shifted toward the red end of the spectrum; otherwise its shape was identical with its match in the dark-adapted eye. In daily life we experience this shift of spectral sensitivity when red flowers grow dark in the dusk at a time when the blue ones still retain their blueness.

These conclusions, based on comparing foveal cone vision with peripherally dominant rod vision in daylight and in the dark, together with less decisive evidence, were collected in the so-called duplicity theory that explains the differences between daylight vision and night vision by the duplex nature—rods and cones—of the retinal receptors. Everything that I have mentioned proved to be fundamental knowledge and theoretically sound when it was analyzed at the retinal level by the potent electrophysiological methods of the present age. Most of the old work was car-

ried out in Germany and was inspired by schools headed by
Purkinje, Aubert, Helmholtz, Hering, König, von Kries,
and, on the photochemical side, by Kühne.[94,95]
Hering more than these other physiologists inclined toward psychological points of view. He defined the pairs of
contrast colors that neutralize each other—such as red-
green and blue-yellow—and ascribed these effects to two
opposite processes. Similarly, the enhancement of white-
ness and blackness by contrast was attributed to the same
opposite processes that were held to be fundamental
neural metabolic events, one breaking down, the other re-
constituting cellular material. Although their names, katabolism and anabolism, mean little to us today, the notion of
two basic opposite processes was destined to live in the
minds of many physiologists and to rise to prominence in
Sherrington's ideas on synaptic excitation and synaptic inhibition as two opposing processes summing algebraically
at the membrane of the neuron.[96]
    Although much more was done in the field of visual psy-
chophysics, what I have mentioned should illustrate the
aims of this science. Inasmuch as physiological explanations were attempted, they referred to the retina as the
only interpretable alternative to phenomenology or sheer
description. Similarly in acoustics, analysis of the sound
waves was shown to be carried out by some kind of resonance mechanism in the cochlea capable of responding differentially to sine waves. By Fourier analysis the sine waves
could be obtained mathematically or, alternatively but less
perfectly, be picked up by resonators such as those
designed for the physiological laboratory by Helmholtz.
The localization of sound by binaural differentiation, just
as binocular localization in space (depth perception),

should be mentioned as important subjects of classical psychophysics.

When today the old stimulus-response psychophysics is being criticized (for example, by Gibson)[97] as providing irrelevant information because animals are interested in objects, places, or events rather than in pure tones or pure spectral lights, this attitude can be defended only if one chooses to neglect the history of our endeavors to understand neural mechanisms. Although it is certainly true that the biological survival value of our sense organs has depended on recognition of objects rather than on purified, isolated stimulus attributes, it is equally true that biological understanding as such has to originate in definitions of a number of simple variables and then proceed to create complex structures of insight on a firm grasp of elementa. The evidence for this statement lies in the usefulness of psychophysical knowledge, demonstrated when advancing electronics made the retina itself accessible to analysis.

I shall give a final example to emphasize what I have said in defense of the psychophysical tradition. By tying the definitions of basic stimulus units of color to spectral lights, it became possible to quantify trichromatic color-matching with the aid of elementary algebra.[98] Clearly such a state of affairs could only signify that somewhere in the biological apparatus sustaining color perception, a trichromatic mechanism had to exist, most likely located in the receptors themselves. Today we know this to be true. Perhaps, in the end, color has little survival value compared with form, but such understanding as is within reach of the human mind has to begin, in reductionist fashion, with isolated cellular units. Our optic nerve after all, contains about a million fibers, not one single cable, and interpretation is organized by many more millions of single cells in the brain. Within the active group of psychophysical experimenters the limitations of their approach was well understood. Hering, for instance, pointed out that the constancy of brightness and size of objects were real facts beyond reach of understanding in terms of psychophysics.[94] He stated that charcoal in sunshine reflects as much light as snow in the dark, yet charcoal is permanently black and snow permanently white. Similarly, objects in a room do not change their apparent size with a change of distance as does the retinal image. Our own hands, whether held near the face or reaching for something at a distance, always retain their apparent size. At present we are at a level of analysis when it is no longer acceptable to refer such facts simply to "experience" as the jack-of-all-trades capable of explaining everything and nothing, and to leave it at that. The modern psychophysics is concerned also with the nature of the complex neural organizations that deal with perceptions as distinct from sensations. The term "perception" is used here to embrace all aspects of organized, conscious interpretation of the external world including objects, space, and movement—in short, to signify also what Gibson meant with his reference to things that have provided survival value to sense organs and sensory organization.

To call this attitude to sensory experience a new or modern psychophysics seems justifiable because the finest achievements of present-day analytical experimentation have once more been based on attempts to discover elementary building blocks of experience, this time, however, in neurophysiological terms. It may seem tempting to explain mechanisms distinguishing, say, an orange from a yellow rubber ball without recourse to tiresome experiments on neural elements of form perception, on color perception, and on circuits integrating information from skin senses and the eye to match it all against memory, but to fall for such temptations means giving up the search for both principles and "hardware" and accepting pure phenomenology. I have no doubt but that something always will be left over for a purely phenomenological and independent science of psychology. The question is merely, At what stage do we give up? How far can we go at the present moment with explanations largely based on the hardware of specific neural mechanisms?

Choice of Levels of Understanding

Before turning to the intricate physiology of elementary visual experience, it is important to recall the conclusion reached in Chapter 1 to the effect that biological explanations are characterized by levels of understanding representing different points of view and often in addition different techniques and terminologies. Anatomy is always in the background, restricted here to cellular organizations and interconnections. Their operations have to be understood in terms of excitation and inhibition, two processes with opposite effects on the cell membrane: excitation depolarizing it, inhibition re- or hyperpolarizing it. Something is then encoded and transmitted to the next locus for transformation by convergent excitatory and inhibitory synapses, and so on to another station, reediting the message by working on it in the same manner. Several such organizations may be piled up in series and in parallel.

When neural operations are approached from the point of view of their relevance for interpretation of the external world, we may or may not be able to make sense out of results in terms of fluctuations of cellular membrane potentials, though ultimately this would be one of our aims. In this situation one does well to remember the analogy with immunology (Chapters 1 and 2), a science in which a magnificent edifice of strictly applicable rules was erected without any knowledge whatsoever of the chemical processes ultimately responsible for them. From these considerations one may inquire into possible principles of interpretation that might be relevant from the teleological viewpoint without imposing the obligation of delving too deeply into the specific electrochemical mechanisms by which a sensible result is achieved. At any rate, it cannot be my aim to do so here.

The Retinal General Organization

In choosing the retina as our model sense organ, we have the advantage of entering the central nervous system by an instrument that itself is a small nervous center, highly elaborated.[99] Developmental anatomy has shown that it has grown out in ontogeny as a vesicle protruding from the brain. Attaching itself to the surface the vesicle has formed the optic cup, lined by the retina with its rods and cones containing photosensitive material. These receptors connect by a synapse to enlongated cells named "bipolars," which in their turn synapse with the ganglion cell whose long axon (nerve fiber) conducts impulses to the next station halfway up the brain to sites reorganizing the message for distribution to the primary visual area in the cerebral cortex and to other places.

Now, if it merely had been a matter of bipolars and ganglion cells the retinal nervous center might have been simple enough to analyze with the aid of localized microelectrodes. There would be a straightforward path upward, and the most important problems would be solved if one succeeded in finding out how many and what kind of receptors were joined to a bipolar cell and how many bipolars to each ganglion cell. There would be combinations of color sensitivities and luminosity sensitivities to elucidate in relation to convergence and to states of dark adaptation (rods) and light adaptation (cones). But the retinal organization is interested in objects and movements: that is, in delivering purposive responses with survival value for the organism. It is to this end that ever-inventive evolution has brought part of the brain itself down to the surface at the front of the body and endowed it with additional cell layers connecting the ingoing paths from the receptors sideways. To the three cells of the direct input—receptors, bipolars, and ganglions—have been added two laterally operating layers of neurons: the horizontal cells at the feet of the receptors and the amacrine cells at the level of bipolars and ganglions. In this manner the grand interplay of excitation and inhibition characterizing the central nervous system has become available at the first site of image formation.

What these lateral connections do depends very much on the nature of the retina, which in its turn is determined by the status of the animal in the vertebrate phylum. The visual world of the frog controls a number of simple acts that have to be well performed. The virtual absence of a cortex makes the animal dependent on analyzing by the retina itself whatever has to be analyzed. Thus, for instance, the frog's retina easily picks up small black objects moving in toward its center. Higher up in the phylum of vertebrates the eyes have shifted from a lateral to a frontal position to allow stereoscopic vision to replace panoramic sight. The number of receptors and optic nerve fibers has increased, thus improving the "grain" of the retinal surface, but its neural mechanisms tend to be more simply organized than they were in the frog. Higher stations have been entrusted with the task of interpreting the visual messages. The biological purpose of this development lies in the fact that the richer the imagery and, above all, the more differentiated the arsenal of actions of an animal, the greater its need for having basic functions elaborated in places where many different channels carrying information can come together. Consider for instance the delicate acts performed by the eye and hand combination, alluded to in Chapter 2. Such acts have required "encephalization" of control.

However, certain principles of retinal processing of light stimuli are common to all animals. Thus, for instance, most nerve fibers from the ganglion cells respond by impulses to both onset and cessation of light; these reactions are generally spoken of as the on-and-off effects, respectively. How can darkening excite? Few if any channels from the receptors through the retina are purely excitatory. An element of inhibition is added, particularly from the lateral connections, and release of inhibition at cessation of illumination excites the system to discharge. One should remember, too, that in the retina, whose thickness at different sections varies from 0.14 to 0.5 mm, the intercellular distances are so short that membrane de- and repolarizations can influence neighboring neurons directly without having had to be transformed into impulses for an axon. The latter transformation takes place mainly in the ganglion cells that dispatch the final message upward. Within the retinal center a re- or hyperpolarization of the membrane of a bipolar or a ganglion cell causes an inhibition, which reverts to excitation when, at cessation of illumination, the membrane swings back in the direction of depolarization. To this principle of operation by opposite changes of potential should be added its utilization by cellular organizations in specific formations, which will be discussed further in later sections. All this is analyzable, provided that the micromethods of physiology are good enough for this aim. Indeed, within the last ten years fine microelectrodes, in the form of glass capillaries whose tips are invisible except at high magnification in a microscope, have been inserted into all types of properly identified retinal neurons for study of their membrane potentials under stimulation.

Because of the way in which the bed of neurons is organized for distribution of inhibition, which here as elsewhere in the central nervous system is the major modeling instrument, the retina can respond to differences in contours and brightness better than to ambient light. The human eye, in particular, which is slowly drifting and constantly executing small but imperceptible movements, is by them geared to produce a lively display of on and off discharges elicited by light-dark-light variations in the surroundings. Thus its most important stimuli are contrast, change, and movement. It makes very little difference whether a change is in the direction of an increase or a decrease of stimulus strength. The essential factor is a shift in the balance between excitation and inhibition. A retina is designed for the purpose of actively scanning the surrounds.

Retina and Optic Nerve of Mammals

It has already been mentioned that the early work on unitary responses in the late thirties emphasized that change, contours, and movement were powerful stimuli enabling an animal to detect such features of the input. Since then, the philosophy of feature detection has become more sophisticated without always convincing the student of this literature that the assumed "detectors" are coded as such in single nerve cells. Just as a musical harmony is analyzed in the brain in its constituent sine waves, so also the perception of an illuminated oblong may not be represented by an "oblong detector" in the retina or at the cortex but on the basis of some mechanism employing quite different constituents.

A unit fiber in the optic nerve accessible to electrical recording represents a number of receptors and laterally acting neurons that have converged toward a single ganglion cell. Within this complex, stimulation elicits excitatory and inhibitory interactions capable of doing something to the quantal absorption of light in the particular receptors by which the unit primarily is activated. The "receptive field" of this cell is organized to pick up cues and one of the most important cues is movement (Hartline).[38] In the retina of the rabbit about one third of the receptive units also respond to direction of movement with a high degree of selectivity (Barlow and Levick).[100] Such units are rare in the retina of the cat in which the indication of direction of movement has been pushed to higher centers. Thus again, more is entrusted to the retina in the less visually developed rabbit. Directional sensitivity to movement is a truly remarkable achievement by the relatively small number of neurons that are hooked up in a receptive field of the rabbit's retina. Somehow the field must be organized asymmetrically to inhibit movement in one direction and facilitate it in the opposite traverse.

It also seems clear that the retina of the cat must be able to handle information in such a way that direction sensitivity to movement later can be created because its existence has been experimentally demonstrated in the cortical visual area. This is true not only of directional sensitivity to movement but also of whatever building blocks a retina has to serve up for further reinterpretation in higher stations. Thus the purpose of the receptive fields is to generate a kind of design that is applicable as a general groundwork for all the elaborations and abstractions that subsequent stations may effectuate. The most common type of receptive field is therefore likely also to be the most versatile in this regard. In mammals this field tends to be circular with a center whose properties are opposite to those of the periphery (Kuffler).[101] It is referred to as the concentric type of receptive field with an on-center off-periphery or off-center on-periphery. In the rabbit's eye about 60 percent of the receptive fields are concentric and the on- and the off-center fields are about equal. In the cat's retina 80 to 90 percent of the fields are concentric with antagonistic properties of center and surround. Lately it has been found that the surround in its turn is surrounded by a zone repeating the properties of the center. This type of organization, which is loaded with inhibition, is clearly well adapted for recording contours and differences of brightness, change, and contrast rather than ambient light.

Finally, it is necessary to think of the retinal receptive fields as overlapping in distribution and as different sizes, in the retina of the cat from 0.5° to 8° in diameter. The fields in the center of an eye are smaller than those in its periphery. Seeing is scanning the environment. As things glide past us, we shift our gaze consciously and automatically. There are vergence movements adjusting our eyes for stereoscopic accuracy. Especially important are slow "drift" and permanent saccadic movements at durations from some 10 to 60 msec and at amplitudes aggregating around 2 to 13 min of angle. If all these movements are compensated by optical means, the artificially stabilized images tend to fade out, thus showing how essential it is that the eyes should move in the way a touch-sensitive hand moves slightly to identify the texture of a surface. A feature of classical psychophysics emphasized the close analogies between retina and skin though, for the latter, interaction begins higher up, in the spinal cord.

We are not aware of the saccadic movements of the eye, but if one gazes at a picture for some time and records the saccades on a stationary film, their quivering staccato movements will be found to have traced the leading contours of the picture (Figure 6.1).[102] The effect of all this scanning of the surrounding world by the moving retina is then dispatched to nonmovable sites in the brain for evaluation. The next major station is in the subcortical brain and is called the "lateral geniculate body." One might have expected the concentric on-off-on fields to have become averaged out at that level into a less differentiated display. But, on the contrary, the concentric pattern is again reestablished. Nothing shows more clearly that it represents a biological asset that cannot be obliterated before its main task has been completed. The retino-geniculo-cortical path is the one best developed in higher mammals like monkey and man. It is the one primarily charged with the final task of interpreting concentric field patterns.

Subcortical Sites

Two intermediate stations on the passage of visual information upward, the geniculate body and the colliculus superior, have been studied a great deal. I shall not discuss the latter beyond mentioning that it is concerned with the control of eye movements and receives direct projections

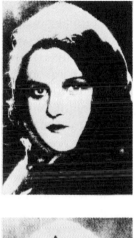

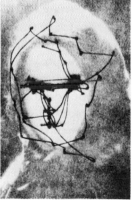

6.1. Photograph of girl's face and record of eye movements during free examination of the photograph with both eyes for one minute. From A. L. Yarbus, *Eye Movements and Vision* (New York: Plenum Press, 1967).

from the slowly conducting optic nerve afferents as well as branches from the fast fibers of the phasic retinal ganglion cells. The colliculus has a precise map of the retina, very large receptive fields, and its cells are directionally sensitive to movement, at least if the fibers descending to it from the cortex are also intact. These findings refer to the cat, in which it seems likely that a general perception of ambient light and discrimination of light intensities is carried out at the collicular level. The colliculus is relatively larger in cats than in primates.

The higher the position of an animal in the vertebrate phylum, the more important becomes the geniculostriate system, the pathway from the geniculate body along the optic radiation fibers to the striate area.[103] ("Striate" is the anatomical name for the primary cortical visual area (numbered 17) that was based on its macroscopic appearance.) The preservation of the concentric type of receptive field in the geniculate body has required some reorganization of the optic nerve fibers because the field boundaries are sharper there than at the retinal level; the fields are smaller, and do not, like their retinal partners, alter in configuration with the state of adaptation. They are, as in the retina, surrounded by an outer rim whose properties repeat those of the center. What has happened is apparently that the new field centers are formed by on-center fibers or off-center fibers. On- and off-center fibers in the optic nerve of the cat are about equally represented among the fastest ones, which are phasic and conduct at rates of 39 meters per second. The fast tonic fibers, conducting at 26 meters per second, were found to be largely on-center.

One should not imagine the geniculate body to be a kind of isolated transmitting station. Other influences play on it, such as fibers controlling the general level of arousal, and it has internuncial inhibitory cells of its own that are likely to be of importance for sharpening its receptive fields.

One of the great achievements of anatomical research established that each neuron in the geniculate body predominantly represents a minute region of the retina. Another feat demonstrated that this nucleus is layered in such a manner as to keep the messages from right and left eye separated and to forward them independently upward in the optic radiation. Because the optic radiation fibers mostly connect the two eyes to a single cell in the cortex, the geniculate body is the last station in which the message from each eye can still be individually influenced—also by nonvisual inputs to it—before binocular treatment of it sets in. Regrettably, there is no clear understanding of when and for what purposes nonvisual inputs become operative although various effects have been described.

The mammalian retina is never silent. There is much spontaneous activity, easily recordable in the ganglions or their axons in the optic nerve, even in complete darkness (Granit).[22] After passage through the geniculate body spontaneous firing is reduced because of inhibitory surround activity. The spontaneous activity surviving passage through the geniculate is not of the random character observed in the optic nerve but is characteristically grouped. Why that should be is not understood from the point of view of function. Basic roles of spontaneous activity are to keep the synaptic apparatus trimmed for use, preventing disuse, and to serve as a background for inhibition.

So far, processing of the visual input has been mainly described in terms that are general enough to be valid for the whole vertebrate phylum. Although some important details will be added, enough has been said to show what it is all about. The purely physiological results are physical, chemical, or organizational but their teleological background is clearly discernible. The role of the physiologist is to elucidate the relevance of the various mechanisms for perception. These neural processes are the physical ingredients of what I have called a new psychophysics. Instead of relating external effects of energy to perception as did classical psychophysics, its modern version is concerned with the internal energy transformations at all intermediary levels from receptors upward. This shift of view is a consequence of the developing electronics that began to influence physiology in the twenties and has been wholly dominating the field ever since.

Trigger Features of the Primary Visual Area

To recall that in the cat a single fiber in the optic radiation reaches 5,000 cells in the visual area is to realize that it will be some time before we can claim that we fully understand the role of the cortex as an interpreter of the input. However, in the last fifteen years significant advances have been made, and principles have emerged that throw light on the kind of building blocks that in some way or other must enter into the final integrations that I have referred to under the term perception. Microelectrodes have been used to record the response of single cortical cells in cats and monkeys. These can be said to have demonstrated that the cells pick up such highly specific cues from the surrounding world as orientation in space of a line, edge, or bar, direction and velocity of movement, and contrast, depth, and color. Although the list could perhaps be expanded, it is of less interest to enumerate hypothetical building blocks of perception than to consider the evidence for some of the ones mentioned. The detector philosophy behind these "trigger" features must not be accepted too readily, because a cellular response to any feature also depends on the kind of stimulus pattern that the experimenter has decided on. Thus in Pasadena, Wiersma, working on the eye of a crayfish while his dog was in the room, noticed that whenever the dog wagged its tail, the fiber below his electrode responded with impulses.[104] This, needless to say, did not establish the presence of a "wagging-tail detector" in the eye of the crayfish.

At the level of the cortex diffuse light is still less of a stimulus than it is in the geniculate body. The majority of cells refuse to respond to illumination as such (Jung)[105] but are readily excited by the pattern they require. The comparatively large evoked potential from the cortex in response to diffuse light may spring from small fibers or from fibers originating in more peripheral parts of the retina.

The messages from the geniculate body are wholly re-edited in the cortex. While these cells still react with on-and-off effects, their response fields have now lost the concentric on- or off-center character. When small bars are put on a screen in front of the eye, they have to be turned round in all directions until the particular orientation is found at which the cortical cell belonging to the correct site on the retinal map will respond. A cell may discharge a few impulses at several angles, but there will be an optimal orientation, a region of the order of 15° in the cat and of 10° in the monkey, within which it will respond vigorously. Tested with small spots instead of bars, these fields are found to be elongated, for instance, with a row of excitatory spots flanked by a parallel inhibitory streak on either or both sides. These cells are sensitive to movement at the slow speeds of 1° to 2° per second in the right relation to their axis of orientation. If a stationary stimulus in the shape of a bar is placed so that it stimulates both the excitatory and inhibitory regions, the cell is silent because of the surround of inhibition. This explains their silence in ambient light. Restricted to either part of the total response region, the stimulus will excite at on or off in its preferred axis orientation. This type of orientation-sensitive cell was called "simple" by Hubel and Wiesel, who discovered it in the early sixties. Simple cells are closest to the cortical input (cortical layer VI). Greater complexity is found in the more superficial layers of the cortex (II and III), in which the neurons also tend to be larger.

The "complex cells" of Hubel and Wiesel behave as if they were composed of the projections of several simple cells. The description of complex cells in the monkey underlines the criterion that there is no separation of receptive fields into excitatory and inhibitory strips. "Whereas for simple cells the position of the stimulus was crucial, in the complex a response was evoked on shining the correctly orientated line on any part of the field or by moving the line over the field" (Hubel and Wiesel, 1968, p. 218).[44,106] These cells also differed from the simple ones in tending to possess spontaneous activity. Within the two "simple" and "complex" categories the responses to direction, speed of movement, and orientation vary more than a schematical description can do justice to. It also seems likely that some complex cells receive a direct input in addition to the one from several simple cells. Other workers have since devoted much time to the study of these two cell types in the visual cortex. A very complete description of striate cells is found in a paper by Bishop, Coombs, and Henry (1971).[107]

Hubel and Wiesel named a third cell type "hypercomplex," but the two types described exemplify the way in which sensory rerepresentation produces highly selective cellular structures whose neurons respond to visual stimuli such as orientation and direction of movement by a spatial organization based on excitation and inhibition. A corresponding cellular specialization was not found in the lateral geniculate body nor is it yet at its final level of development in these primary projections to the visual area 17. This is but one stage in a cascading visual interpretation of form, providing cues for direction, edges, movement, and velocity.

Organization within the Visual Cortex

As mentioned in Chapter 4, the retinal surface is localized on the striate area (area 17) as a cellular surface with a high degree of magnification in the foveal region, used for optimal focused vision and a lessening of magnification toward the periphery. This map represents the fundamental positional variable; analysis in terms of single cells (Hubel and Wiesel) disclosed two other organizations grafted upon this basic cartographic design.[106] One is a columnar arrangement found when the microelectrodes were pushed further in at right angles to the cortical surface layers.[44] Within any one column the cells turned out to possess much the same axis of orientation, as if they had formed a little organ within the greater organ to respond to this particular trigger feature. Columns of both simple cells and complex cells were noted. A similar vertical organization had been seen by Mountcastle and Powell studying the somatic sensory cortex.[108] In this cortical region the columns represented different subgroups of such modalities as light touch, deep pressure, and joint.

This kind of orderliness fell into line with the classical

anatomical findings of Ramón y Cajal who emphasized the vertical or, rather, radial direction of cellular organization in the cortex, as did later Lorente de Nó.[108] In the monkey some 18 to 20 possible orientations are represented in the orientation columns, which more accurately are described as thin vertical sheets or cylinders about 0.025 mm wide. There seems to be little if any cross-talk between the orientation columns. Probably their independence is caused by a mechanism of lateral inhibition.

More recently the same authors have found another kind of columnar arrangement based on a variable ocular dominance in cells with binocular projections; most of the cells were found to have projections from both eyes, generally with one or the other eye giving a larger response and thus being the dominant one. Two variables in the ocular dominance columns correspond to the 18 to 20 variables of the orientation columns. These express relative amount of right and left eye contribution to the neuron recorded from. The ocular dominance columns are 0.25 to 0.5 mm across. The orientation and ocular dominance columns are mutually independent, though overlapping textures. Neither type of column is distributed across the visual area in a wholly haphazard manner. It is easily understood that, if orientation columns really are delivering cues for orientation, the basic topographical representation of the retina requires that all orientational subgroups be found within a very small region; otherwise different retinal regions would specialize on different orientations! By using both perpendicular and tangential penetrations in the visual area of the monkey, Hubel and Wiesel have demonstrated that the 18 to 20 orientation variables make a full 180° turn within 0.5 to 1 mm, thus forming, as it were, a new hierarchical "hypercolumn" to deal with this particular parameter. In thinking of such facts one should remember that we see with a moving eye. In an ocular dominance column each cell responds to corresponding sites in the two eyes. If these are separately tested, the stimuli have to be similarly orientated. Just as the orientation columns are grouped into a hypercolumn taking care of the whole array of orientation variables, so the ocular dominance columns produce a complete left-right to right-left eye dominance turn within a hypercolumn whose size appears to be identical with that representing the 18 to 20 orientations. Such hypercolumns are likely to be organizational units, dealing with both orientation and binocularity.

Contrast and Spatial Frequency

Under contrast and spatial frequency falls work that also has led to singularly interesting psychophysical correlations.[109] The results refer to new methods of studying contrast by gratings of dark and light stripes. By electronic methods, gratings with rectangular or sinusoidal alternating dark and bright parallels can be conveniently produced to be viewed on a television screen. Any desirable spatial repetition frequency in cycles per degree of visual angle can be obtained at any chosen degree of contrast. The definition of contrast is the difference between the maximal and minimal luminosities of the dark and bright stripes, that is $L_{max} - L_{min}$, divided by their sum, $L_{max} + L_{min}$. The mean luminosity, which is this value divided by 2, can be kept constant despite variations in spatial frequency and contrast. In this arrangement the stimulus is contrast at a defined spatial frequency, not luminosity (brightness as such). The results are mostly given in terms of sensitivity to contrast, which is the inverse value of the contrast required for a constant criterion response. With this technique it is possible to study (1) the response of single cells, (2) an assembly of such cells eliciting an evoked cortical potential, and (3) the subjective response of human subjects. This multiplicity of approach is one of its major attractions.

Beginning with the retinal ganglion cells in the cat, it is found that different cells are set to preferential spatial frequencies of the grating. In the retina the selectivity is not very high, but it is increased in the lateral geniculate body, and in the "simple" cells of the primary visual area sensitivity is further sharpened to spatial frequencies. The complex cell types in the cortex of the cat are less sharply tuned to specific spatial frequencies. The general conclusion from this work (Campbell, Enroth-Cugell, Fiorentini, Maffei, Robson) is that the geniculostriate system of the highly developed mammals possesses channels that serve as spatial frequency analyzers in combination with spatial orientation. The gratings have to be turned to the right orientation of the cortical cell tested for spatial frequency detection.

A way of linking these experiments to psychophysics proved to be the phenomenon of selective adaptation to spatial frequency as utilized by Campbell and Kulikowski, and Blakemore and Campbell.[109] Light from a grating was split by a prism into two beams, one of which could be rotated in its plane. When at verticality the rotating grating was exactly superposed on its partner, a masking effect of selective adaptation depressed the sensitivity to contrast. As the rotating companion was turned round, the masking effect was reduced—at 12° to either side by as much as a factor of 2.

In the continuation of this work a sinusoidal grating was

used that stimulated by being alternated in phase by 180°
eight times a second. Neither contrast nor average luminance is altered by the phase shift. The gaze was allowed to
wander freely to prevent formation of afterimages. In this
manner there was first established the distribution curve of
contrast sensitivity for a range of spatial frequencies (Figure 6.2). Then selective effects were introduced by pre-
adapting to different spatial frequencies, which were
found to give narrow bands of depression of contrast sensitivity (Figure 6.3). The sinusoidal frequencies used for adaptation are found above the curves. There is a lower limit
of about 3 cycles per degree to the existence of specific frequency channels. Their full range is about 3 to 4 octaves,
one octave being a change in spatial frequency by a factor
of 2. All bands of these spatial-frequency channels were
found to be of much the same width, even when an increase of contrast was used to augment the adaptive effect
in absolute values. The bandwidth has since been shown to
be even narrower than indicated by this method. Maffei
and Fiorentini have since found in kittens kept in the dark
a lasting selective depression to a spatial frequency of 0.45
cycle per degree of visual angle to which the animals were
exposed two to three hours daily for two and one-half to
three months.[110]

Stimulation by alternating phase shifts of 180° within a
frequency pattern is a method that also lends itself to application in connection with a summation technique for recording evoked potentials. The recording electrode is over
the occipital region of the skull, using an averaging computer which by electronic summation adds the responses
from 200 sweeps within each of which the individual
evoked potential is too small to rise above the noise level.
This electronic summation technique has been used with

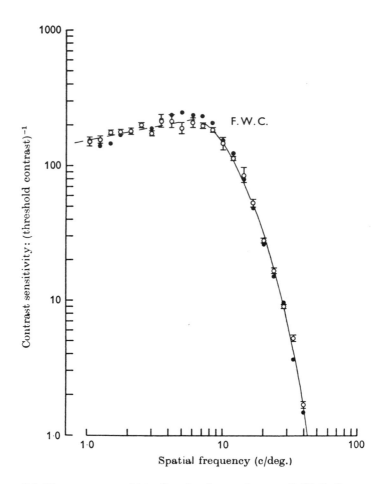

6.2. The contrast sensitivity function for an observer, F. W. C. Contrast sensitivity is plotted on an arbitrary logarithmic scale against spatial frequency. The open circles and vertical bars show initial threshold estimates with 1 S.E. (n = 6). The filled circles are repeat determinations at the end of the series of adaptation experiments. The continuous curve is the function e^{-f} and the interrupted portion was fitted by eye to the low frequency data points. During threshold determinations the pattern was turned on and off twice per second, without changing mean luminance. From C. Blakemore and F. W. Campbell, *J. Physiol. (Lond.)* 203 (1969):237–260.

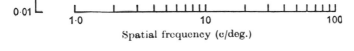

6.3. Adaptation characteristics derived as in 6.2 for five adapting spatial frequencies. Each arrow marks the frequency of adaptation and above it is the symbol used for the relative threshold elevation caused by the adaptation. Points are joined in order of spatial frequency. The adapting frequencies were 3.5, 5.0, 7.1, 10.0, and 14.2. From C. Blakemore and F. W. Campbell, *J. Physiol. (Lond.)* 203 (1969):237–260.

both animals and man. The amplitude of the evoked potential is found to be proportional to the apparent contrast. This amplitude from a low-contrast grating is markedly reduced or virtually obliterated by preadaptation to a high-contrast grating of the same mean luminance. By this method there has also been found selective adaptation to spatial frequencies.

The Role of Spatial Frequency Channels

Most interesting is that the psychophysical approach and the recording of evoked potentials bridge the gap to the results obtained with single cortical cells. This means that the "language" of cellular responses in impulses per second can be generalized by Fourier analysis of spatial frequency channels carrying sine waves.[111] The importance of this approach is that Fourier analysis is a very general mathematical tool. It is not necessary to use a sinusoidal variation of contrast. A square wave, for instance, can be considered as the sum of a series of sine wave components whose frequencies are odd multiples of the fundamental frequency. Or the easily produced sawtooth wave can be used. In both cases it has been shown that the amplitude of its fundamental sine component is the decisive one for the measured psychophysical effect.

There is interocular transfer of the selective adaptation to spatial frequency just as there is the well-known interocular transfer in color matching: green light into one eye and red into the other makes the subject synthesize yellow. Maffei and Fiorentini showed that if the fundamental sine wave of a square wave pattern is shone into one eye and its third harmonic—the largest one—into the other, the observer actually sees a square.[111] In this respect the eye behaves like the ear, which analyzes a sound into its sine wave components, the pure tones. These have been found localized on the auditory cortex in a spatial pattern reminiscent of a xylophone.

To sum up with a quotation from Campbell and Robson (1968), the eye uses several independent "detector mechanisms, each preceded by a relatively narrow-band filter 'tuned' to a different frequency."[109] Each filter has its own contrast-sensitivity function. Their envelope is the contrast-sensitivity function of the visual system of man illustrated in Figure 6.2.

The comparison with the acoustic system suggests that a mechanism based on analyzing visual images by means of independent channels of spatial frequencies would render the absolute size of the retinal image negligible for its recognition. Just as a musical interval (frequency ratio) can be identified independently of its position in the auditory spectrum, so also can a seen object be identified by the frequency ratios of the channels by which it is interpreted in the cortex. "Only the harmonic content would have to be stored in the memory system and this would require a much smaller store than if the appearance of every familiar object had to be learned at every common magnification. This generalization for size, and therefore distance, would greatly facilitate the process of learning to recognize images in their natural environment" (Blakemore and Campbell, 1969, p. 258).[109] The orientationally selective channels would impose the restriction that recognition of familiar, complex objects have to be seen at the orientation at which they were learned. The evidence for this, they say, is

HERE IS THE EVIDENCE

The conclusion is that we cannot generalize for orientation the way we do for magnification. If one draws two identical squares but places one of them standing on a corner, it will look more like a diamond (Rock) than a square.[112] In man there is orientational preference for the vertical and horizontal directions. While the resolving power for gratings is at a frequency of 35.5 cycles per degree of visual angle for these two directions, it is between 25.5 and 29 cycles per degree for oblique gratings.

These experiments, conclusions, and suggestions clearly illustrate trends in the modern version of psychophysics. Its classical counterpart could register great achievements, but it had little success with problems of form perception and contrast. The development of electronics is at the back of the striking progress in understanding processing of visual information. The aim has been to discover building blocks of perception, cortical detectors of characteristic features, or hidden detectors like the spatial frequency channels.

It would be premature to hazard a guess as to how many detectors there might be. There may be some based on the subdivision of the fast retinal fibers into phasic (transient) and tonic (sustained).[113] This is suggested by the difference in the perceived threshold for flicker and for pattern recognition. The phasic ones might record flicker, the tonic ones contrast. But, as previously emphasized, some caution is always indicated in ascribing new, specific detector properties to the system merely because it can differentiate one thing from another. Are there, for instance, detectors for bar width? This has been proposed, but one would expect some degree of selective adaptation to bar width if this feature were separately channeled. Such an effect has not been found and so, for the time being, it seems sufficient to

make detection of bar width dependent on the spatial frequency channels. It is not necessary to think of all channels
for orientation and spatial frequency as rigidly fixed. The
experiments mentioned in Chapter 3 dealt with means of
influencing evoked potentials as indicators of an altered
sensitivity to verticality. It is a moot question what is
laid down genetically and within what limits adaptability is
available   to   counteract   genetical   rigidity   (compare
Chapter 3).[114]

Some Cues for Stereopsis

Stereopsis or stereoscopic vision means the capacity to perceive depth and solidity. Its basic prerequisite is frontal
placement of the eyes causing overlap of the right and left
visual fields. The same image is seen from slightly different
points of view in binocular parallax. Because the two hemispheres of the brain are interconnected and half of the optic nerve fibers from each eye cross over to join those of the
other eye in the striate area of the opposite cortex, the two
eyes can serve as a single, cortical cyclopean eye.

   If one focuses the gaze on a finger held at a convenient
reading distance, a finger of the other hand at some distance directly behind it appears doubled. If the gaze is
shifted to the distant finger, the one closer to the eyes
is seen doubled. The images in focus have fallen on corresponding points of the two retinas. Points that do not correspond are disparate. At a certain degree of disparity
the two images glide apart instead of fusing into one. In
classical psychophysics and ophthalmology much work was
devoted to elucidating depth perception in relation to disparity, correspondence, and the size of the fusional area.
In addition to binocular parallax other cues aid us in per-

ceiving depth, even monocularly, as known by painters for centuries.

As we have seen, most cells in the primary visual area could be stimulated from either eye, provided that similar trigger features (orientation, in the first instance) were used for stimulating their corresponding points, one eye tending to be dominant and elicit a larger cortical discharge. These observations set the stage for studying the implications of correspondence and disparity at the cortical level (Barlow, Blakemore, Pettigrew).[115] The basic contention is that cat and man, both with frontally placed eyes and a well-developed geniculostriate system, possess essentially similar mechanisms of stereoscopic vision, though man, a skillful toolmaker, probably developed them for greater precision in near vision.

If disparity were a cue to fusion and stereopsis, it would have to be somehow signaled in experiments with a binocularly excitable neuron under the microelectrode. The stimulus would be a slit moving over the receptive field at the correct orientation. The experiment would begin by ascertaining the responses of the two eyes separately. Aligned for stimuli in precise correspondence, the cell would generally sum up their effects. The images would then be moved apart horizontally by a prism in the light beam. This is equivalent to testing disparities by shifting the image of each eye toward or away from the focus in imitation of convergence or divergence movements of the eye bulbs. The experimental question is, How does the binocular neuron, which responds optimally at correspondence, behave in slight disparity?

It was found that (in the cat) a departure from correspondence by as little as 2 to 3 minutes of arc causes an inhibition of the neuronal response. This figure for sensitivity to misalignment refers to the center of the eye and to neurons with both simple and complex response fields. In man the accuracy in foveal vision is about ten times greater, but then, to judge from work on monkeys, his foveal receptive fields would also be smaller than those of the cat. But even when one eye elicited a much larger response than the other, the binocular response was heavily suppressed if its weaker partner was projected in slight disparity, indeed, as heavily as to be smaller than the monocular response at nonoptimal disparity.

The role of the hypercolumn representing right-left to left-right ocular dominance in stereopsis is not yet fully clarified, but it seems that with a slightly moving eye the fluctuations in ocular dominance within it must be of considerable importance as cues for depth and solidity. The eyes search for the optimal binocular response and are guided by the fact that, for instance, a left-eye target evokes a higher sensitivity to orientation than its right partner or the opposite. But even if we do not yet possess a complete understanding of how the cues for stereopsis are built up, the facts referred to must be of eminent importance. At the next level in the parastriate areas (18 and 19), these cues complete their specifications, as shown by the most recent results of Hubel and Wiesel with neurons in area 18 of the monkey. Some of them merely respond when the target is at a definite distance from the eye.

Orientation-selectivity of binocular neurons in the cat may vary a great deal for the two eyes; within a range of more than 15° at a standard deviation of 6° to 9°, as found by Blakemore and by Fiorentini and Maffei. This raises the question as to what feature in depth perception might be served by the need for binocular precision in selectivity to orientation as an additional cue. The experiments of these authors suggested that neurons with different preferred orientations in the two eyes would respond best to the contours of objects tilted about the horizontal axis toward, or away from, the animal's eyes. In the previous section it was shown that visual objects are analyzed into spatial sine waves that are channeled independently to the cortex along bands of increasingly narrower width. Fiorentini and Maffei (1971), turning to a psychophysical study of gratings of different spatial frequencies, found that (1) two vertical gratings of the same spatial frequencies, presented stereoscopically, gave a fused binocular image in the frontal plane but that (2) if they were of different frequencies, the binocular image appeared to be tilted with that side farther away from the eye whose spatial frequency was the higher.[115] Reversing the spatial frequencies for the two eyes reversed the tilt. Inclinations of 30° and 40° were obtained with frequency differences of 8 and 12 percent respectively. Translating this experiment into recording of evoked potentials, Fiorentini and Maffei found that the binocularly tilted images, caused by gratings of different frequencies for the two eyes, gave larger evoked potentials than those of equal spatial frequency that stereoscopically appeared to be in the same plane.

The search for cues for stereoscopic vision is a field in the making and still expanding. The results mentioned here merely indicate its complexity and contact with other detector problems previously discussed.

Feature Detection and Perception

It would be a cardinal mistake to assume that "feature detectors" or for that matter "featureless detectors," such as spatial sine wave frequencies within a complex figure, are building blocks of perception in any other sense than as neural organizations making available "cues" for a central "interpreter" capable of matching them against other frameworks of reference. Perceptual interpretation is by no means restricted to the striate area (17) or even to surrounding parastriate areas (18 and 19) concerned with vision. Distortions of visual space are seen in patients with a lesion elsewhere in the brain interfering with interaction between sensory modalities. Perception of verticality may be disturbed in cerebellar lesions. Bender and Diamond state that defects in vestibulo-ocular mechanisms may cause gross optical illusions. They have had patients in whom "the entire visual field is skewed or even inverted so that the examiner may appear to be upside down and standing on the ceiling" (p. 181).[116]

Then there is the whole range of invariance phenomena—constant size, movement, velocity, color; there are the ambiguous figures and an ever-increasing number of visual illusions, all of which provide glimpses of how different or equivocal features are interpreted on the basis of established frameworks of reference, as yet hardly translatable into "hardware." For this purpose—a goal not entirely out of reach—it is commendable to bear in mind two essential principles: (1) the brain is capable of using every possible "cue," should this be required, to hunt for the most sensible conclusion that can be drawn from available information and retained knowledge; and (2) because the eyes are in continuous movement, it is not possible to think in terms of unitary "detectors" without realizing that evaluation of them for percepts and action mostly is based on large numbers of such cells.

The old physiologists discussed perception without

knowing that counteraction of eye movements by optical correction makes the image fade out. This discovery is relatively recent (Riggs, Ratliff, Cornsweet, and Cornsweet; Ditchburn).[117] For technical reasons experimental work on single cells is restricted to a steady eye, but in actual life the relevant cues are multicellular and overlapping, and so it is quite likely that essential components of feature detection or perhaps aspects of interaction between already known detectors have been missed in the physiological experiments reviewed. The many unexpected revelations made by application of a spatial-frequency variation emphasize this point.

The difficulties facing the psychology of perception in relation to known physiological mechanisms of feature extraction are well illustrated by what is thought and written about the perceptions of movement and size constancy. The question that has evoked the greatest interest in this connection is why the external world does not move at all despite the perennial scanning of it by eye movements. Mostly voluntary sweeps of the eye over the environment have been considered. We know that the external world moves if one pushes the eye bulb.

The physiologist would begin by asking whether there is any possible cue for stability of the external world. His first answer would come from the experiments of Wurtz on the cortex of the cat.[118] The animal was trained to make horizontal 20° eye movements and 188 neurons in its striate cortex were studied. Of them 48 percent did not respond at all when the eye moved rapidly over the stimulus, which was a slit of optimal orientation for the neuron isolated. Thus the majority of the cells indicated that the external world is steady. Two other types of cell recorded movement of the stimulus. One type, 32 percent of the total, was excited; the other, 20 percent, was inhibited by movement of the slit. All 188 cells fired in response to a stationary stimulus if the latter was adjusted to the right orientation. The brain is faced with the task of sorting out the significance of these messages in relation to eye movements (saccadic and oscillatory ones, drifts and voluntary movements) and to objects moving against a steady background; in other words, to develop appropriate frameworks of reference. These are not established by purely visual means. We know the orientation-sensitive cells to be influenced by somatic and vestibular inputs. These help in differentiating the stable world from moving objects. The experiments on inversion lenses and prismatic goggles mentioned in Chapter 3 show that new frameworks of reference can be established within hours, days, or weeks. A much longer time has been available for the developing brain to pick up and learn to evaluate the large number of cues differentiating between a stable world and objects moving past the retina. Messages from the eye muscles can hardly be neglected in this connection.

Two hypotheses have dealt with cues related to eye muscles. Helmholtz assumed that the commands to the eye muscles were also dispatched to the sites perceiving movement, thereby implying that motor efferent impulses could stabilize the seen world by a kind of cancellation of the perception of movement. This would explain that passive pushing on the eye bulb makes the world move, while movements controlled by eye muscles keep it steady. Sherrington thought of a similar role for sensory impulses from the eye muscles, a more attractive proposition. Neither of them, of course, knew about the differentiating messages from the retina to cortical cells (Wurtz),[118] nor did they know that the eye muscles of man are particularly well provided with muscle spindles (Cooper and Daniel),[119] which are sense organs adjustable in sensitivity from the brain by special motor nerves. The spindles are activated by commands from the brain and are capable of feeding back information on eye movements. As therefore an afferent apparatus, specifically activated by its own motor fibers, exists for delivering the information that the eye muscles are active, it seems unnecessary to postulate a special informative role for other efferent motor impulses, an idea that raises the obvious question of why then any muscular sense organs? It has actually been shown that, in the absence of other cues, we are able to use these endings to gauge the direction of our gaze in the dark (Skavenski).[120] Normally an ample supply of cues would make perception of muscular impulses superfluous. But they could contribute information to the automatic selection among frameworks of reference.

In the end, perception involves an instant conclusion as to what is what by an "interpreter" in the brain, and this, as we shall see, involves coactivation of the large portions of the cortex that so far have been left aside. At this point it is pertinent again to recall the warning of Berzelius not to advance explanations for what cannot be explained at a given moment. It is best to admit straight away that the elusive, mostly automatized processes interpreting the external world still belong to the many well-kept secrets of a brain designed to create frameworks of reference for stability and invariance. What ultimately becomes a conscious percept is but one tenth of an iceberg riding on its nine submerged fractions. Despite this, it is always necessary to go as far as possible in looking for guiding principles in the creation of such frameworks of reference for the act of interpretation, as I shall do now in briefly considering illusions and invariance phenomena. The Pulfrich effect is a well-known illusion.[121] A pendulum is swung in a vertical plane facing an observer who has covered one eye with a gray glass. He then sees the pendulum swinging in a circle whose plane is horizontal. This stereoscopic illusion is held to be cued by the difference in latent period of arrival of the signals from the two differentially illuminated eyes. A decrease of stimulus intensity lengthens the latent period; hence the signal from the darkened eye will be delayed relative to that of the other eye. There may be additional cues from the organizations for the perception of depth.

When driving in the dark beside a forest as a child, I saw for the first time the well-known and impressive phenomenon of the moon gliding forward along the treetops, in my case at the speed of the horse, slow or fast depending on the road. In this example the moon was perceptually at the treetops and should therefore soon be left behind the moving vehicle. In reality the moon was very far away so that its image on the retina was of constant size at a constant site. The "interpreter" in the brain, matching input against experience, faces this conflict of information, and, very sensibly, concludes that an apparent image at the treetops, which does not remain behind the moving vehicle, itself must be moving with the speed of the latter. Again characteristically seen movement is a conclusion based on an established framework of reference. Similarly the stroboscopic perception of movement is a conclusion. None of these illusions can be dependent on information from eye muscles. Yet in no way do they differ from "legitimate," seen movements.

The most general lesson from such observations is that we must not underestimate what the interpreting brain itself adds to make the seen world more intelligible than does a pure peripheral input, dependent though the cortex is on information from feature detectors. The purposive brain requires a considerable degree of invariance, size constancy,[122] a fixed verticality, approximately invariant surface colors, some constancy of velocity and direction of movement and, above all, a steady world; in short, a large number of what one is fully entitled to call "reliable illusions." They are all constant errors with respect to the informational content of the primary sensory message. A world in which, for instance, my hands all the time varied in size with the retinal image would be intolerable! And so the brain does what no computer can imitate: in growing and developing, it creates the world it needs. This purposive process has led to the automatic, fast inferences by which sensory information is compared with relevant frameworks of reference for the most plausible end result.

Cues, Detectors, and Sites of Interpretation

I have not treated the terms "cue" and "feature detector" as synonyms but rather as overlapping in meaning without being identical. Against the background of the many examples given, it is now possible to differentiate the two terms from the point of view of their contribution to "explanation." Cue is the more general term. When the Pulfrich illusion is explained by the difference in latent period of the two eyes or when, similarly, the time difference between the arrival of sounds at the two ears provides an important cue to the localization of sound, no definite neural "likeness" is envisaged between "cue" and "percept"; there is nothing in the nature of the cue to explain the psychological end result of its operation. Only a causal relationship is assumed. The term "feature detector" goes a step farther. It signifies that a particular neural organization, generally localized anatomically, presents features serving a specified purpose defined psychologically. Thus orientation-sensitivity of a column of cortical neurons is believed to fulfill the purpose of making it possible for the organism to detect the orientation of contours. The orientation of the cortical response field is given the psychologically defined purpose of serving as a building block for a percept. This type of conceptualization is strongly rooted in teleology. The psychological act of perceiving need not itself be—and from what we know is not—localized to the striate area. The detected features in their turn become cues for further processing.

The finding of cortical neurons representing different orientations could alternatively be interpreted as a consequence of a wholly nonpurposive chance recombination of fibers from the concentric field as mapped out on the geniculate body. With each optic radiation fiber distributing terminals to 5,000 neurons in the cortex, absence of orientational selectivity would perhaps be more surprising than its presence. Chance would see to that. The role of orientational selectivity as a feature detector is a hypothesis—but a very attractive one—that implies that the orientation-sensitive arrangement is purposive from the biological point of view. Its columnar organization fully supports this hypothesis as against pure chance. One of its attractions lies in the directness by which the experimental observations are translated into psychology. For those who despise teleological thinking, orientation-selectivity will still

remain an interesting finding, though inexplicable even in the less specific sense of a cue.

The same kind of teleological directness is not found in the hypothesis explaining sensitivity to contrast and contours by spatial sine wave channels of upward increasing narrowness of bandwidth. Some might prefer to call this postulate a cue rather than a feature detector. My own preference is for interpreting it as a feature-detecting device, probably the most fundamental one when form is concerned. If one inquires after the biological asset contained in the elaboration of concentric on-off fields and their maintenance up to the level of the geniculate body, the discovery of spatial frequency channels would seem to contain an essential component of the answer, synthesizing as they do sensitivity to edges, contrast, and orientation. Sine wave channeling need not for that reason be the absolute prerogative of the geniculostriate system. Visual messages also enter the brain through other inputs. These may work in the same general way, only in a less perfect manner. Much recent evidence indicates that in some mammals brightness and patterns can be discriminated in the absence of the striate area (Doty; Weiskrantz).[123]

The first unitary feature detector ever described in the visual sphere was embodied in the experimental demonstration (1939) that some afferent fibers from the retinas of frogs and snakes only responded to restricted regions of the spectrum.[22] These feature detectors were very narrow bands of color sensitivity whose existence recently again has been confirmed in the frog.[124] Next a demonstration in goldfish showed that contrast colors were antagonistically coupled by a mechanism that seemed to involve interaction in horizontal cells (McNichol and Svaetichin).[125] Specific color sensitivity appears to be best developed in the surrounding region called the prestriate cortex. Columnar organizations of neurons have been found that represent very narrow bands of specific color sensitivity. Apart from color the exact stimulus requirements of individual neurons varied. Some units responded optimally to particular shapes at particular orientations with color sensitivity added as a requirement. Other neurons were merely color-sensitive. Some units had both surround and successive color contrast (Zeki).[126] Such "higher" integrations will be discussed in Chapter 9.

The first lesson that can be drawn from the early results concerns encephalization. The extremely narrow bands of wavelength specificity found in the retinas of frogs and snakes in the monkey occur in the lateral geniculate body[127] and in the prestriate cortex. The next lesson is that fundamentally the process of interpretation is built up stepwise to increasingly higher degrees of specification. In the present example neurons in the prestriate area combined properties of different feature detectors, suggesting that specification has to precede synthesis, thus justifying the search for feature detectors even when their survival value may not be immediately evident. The primary or striate area (17) delivers "features" to the adjacent areas (18 and 19). In this manner rerepresentation can lead to a synthetic combination of features within the function of a single neuron. This processing of information does not end in the prestriate area. Nor is it necessarily true that information only spreads vertically and horizontally within the purely cortical bed of neurons.

Much research today is centered on a visual region in primates called the inferotemporal area, which need be known merely as a portion of cortex in the lower temporal part of the brain (see Figures 4.3 and 4.4). Attention was drawn to this region in 1954 (Mishkin and Pribram).[128] Lesions there interfere with visual discrimination even when the visual fields for all appearances are intact. The kind of discrimination that is disturbed involves visual choice procedures requiring learning. Difficulties of visual form recognition have been noted in human beings with inferotemporal lesions, suggesting that higher grades of abstraction take place in the inferotemporal brain. There are transcortical paths to this region from the striate and prestriate areas, and it has efferent connections to several subcortical nuclei. I mention the inferotemporal region here merely to indicate the existence of frontiers of knowledge about building blocks of perception going beyond those to which this chapter has been devoted (see also Chapter 9).

7
Birth and Some Consequences of the Single-Cell Approach to Problems of Motor Control

Muscle moves the world.

What To Explain

Our explanations in this field are not tied to conscious awareness the way they were in dealing with perception. Many most delicate and carefully adjusted movements need be performed under the full blaze of consciousness, at least during an initial period of practice. As a rule they do not require it in the long run. Postural changes—essentially adjustments to gravity—are continuously in operation without ever being attended to. And several well-known reflexes, such as the knee jerk, elicited by the physician's hammer for diagnostic purposes, or limb withdrawal in response to pain, are completed before we have had time to take notice of them. Most voluntary acts are merely "triggered" by willing, triggered in the sense that the act is voluntarily demanded but then accomplished automatically.

Once more all this shows that conscious awareness is an independent process *sui generis,* also that even the most detailed knowledge about the motor mechanisms never can help us to understand consciousness. We can only attempt to understand the organization of motor acts or, at least, some of their essential boundary conditions. We came a little closer to consciousness in searching for building blocks of perception in the previous chapter. There were after all results that could be hypothetically explained as leading up to conscious percepts. Then what is the aim of scientific work in the motor field? Or, in other words, What do we want to explain? What is the nature of "explanation" in this case?

An essential point to remember is that the movement itself is the interpreter, either of a sensory input or of something stored that emerges as a voluntary or automatic analyzable act. This means that the element of purposiveness and thus of prediction is very much in the foreground in the motor field, so much so that nonpurposive movements tend to be regarded as outright pathological. A prolific line of motor research therefore deals with teleological questions: what is the purpose of a reflex; why is a movement preferentially tonic or phasic; what is its aim, does it serve running, walking, or standing; why do eyes move and what is the role of eye movements in perception. These are specimens of why questions requiring answers. Sherrington used the term "integration" to mean interaction of nervous pathways for a definite purpose.[96] But most of the work in this field is not concerned with such purely teleological questions but with the composite problems of how motor mechanisms are purposively organized; that is, interaction itself, the role of different cortical, subcortical, cerebellar, and spinal sites, in controlling and initiating movement, how sense organs operate reflexes, what "feedback" signifies in the regulation of motor acts, to what extent movements are preprogrammed and independent of constant or intermittent feedback, and so on.

I emphasized that a movement embodies a purposive interpretation in objective terms, for instance, of a sensory input that can be shown to be its cause. This is particularly true of the spinal reflexes, and for this very reason the whole modern approach to the study of the intricate mechanisms of the central nervous system, which is based on understanding synaptic action, arose out of reflexology as utilized analytically by Sherrington. His concepts evolved into many explanations of the nature of the neural events responsible for observable interactions between sensory channels capable of initiating or suppressing reflex movements.[129] This was the work of a lifetime, hardly compressible to the extent required here, but I shall try to indicate by using a simple experiment on spinal reflexes how some of Sherrington's—and thus our own—major concepts were derived.

The Reflex: Its Use and Limitations

Openly or implicitly all experimentation with spinal reflexes presupposes the existence of a "wiring diagram," the reflex arc, and development in this field has been much concerned with making such diagrams more detailed and more precise. Sherrington's active period (about 1895 to 1935) coincided roughly with that of the Spanish anatomist Ramón y Cajal (1852–1934) who provided the basic wiring diagrams that until then had been missing. "He solved at a stroke," said Sherrington, "the great question of the direction of the nerve-currents in their travel through brain and spinal cord," proving that it was unidirectional, and thus afferent (sensory), efferent (motor) in the reflex arc and, in between the two, based on synaptic contacts between neurons. At an early date Sherrington accepted the notion that information is transmitted by such contacts between nerve cells. He did this by introducing the term "synapse" in 1897, before the full histological evidence for the neuron theory—a cellular contact theory—was available and while many workers still believed that at the central end there was a kind of protoplasmic continuum of cellular material.[129]

In the present era of electronics, microelectrodes, microchemistry, and electron microscopy the synapse is a familiar object of study from many points of view in many laboratories, but how was it to be approached when the indicator of the postulated synaptic activity had to be a reflex muscular contraction? The reply to this question is based on a type of experiment in which the reflex contraction of a mechanically freed muscle is recorded "isometrically." This term was introduced in the last century by Adolf Fick (1829–1901) and means that the muscle is prevented from shortening so that the whole contractile effect emerges as gram tension, recordable by a tension-sensitive myograph.[130] The input to the spinal cord is provided by stimulation of sensory nerves or their end organs.

The central issue in this type of classical experiment concerns interaction between excitation and inhibition.[131] Assume that each cell in a pool of neurons with axons innervating a given muscle receives convergent projections of synapses from afferent nerve fibers (input)A, B, and C. Proceeding to stimulate these nerves individually by repetitive electrical shocks one would, for instance, find A yielding 500 gram reflex tension of the muscle, B 1,000 gram, and C no effect whatsoever. We know that the muscle's motor nerve stimulated by itself, that is directly, not reflexly, raises 3,000 gram tension. Thus A and B have only elicited fractional effects. They have not succeeded in eliciting discharges from all the neurons of the muscle. When we stimulate the two afferent nerves A and B together, we obtain 2,800 gram tension, or a great deal more than their sum (1,500 gram).

The explanation of this experiment is that A and B also had a subthreshold fringe of overlapping excitatory effects on the pool. Neither afferent nerve by itself could raise these weakly excited neurons to firing level. With this conclusion we have also introduced the concept of a graded excitatory state or level of excitability whose duration can be tested by stimulating with A and B sequentially at varying intervals from complete temporal overlap to any desirable degree of separation. Next, A, B, and C are stimulated together. This only produces 200 gram tension or even less than A had given alone. This result is interpreted to mean that nerve C has inhibitory synapses on the cells of the motoneuron pool of the tested muscle, indeed, enough of them to cancel much of the excitation.

By experiments of this general type it could be shown that excitation E and inhibition I are graded states of opposite character, capable of what looked like algebraic summation of opposites (plus and minus signs) when they clashed on the same neuronal membrane. The necessary evidence for precise algebraic summation of reflexes has since been given by extra- and intracellular methods in the author's laboratory.[37]

With muscle tension the index of E or I, the neuron on which these influences converge is the motor horn cell or motoneuron whose axon serves as the "final common path" (Sherrington), distributing its branches to end plates (synapses) on a number of individual muscle fibers. The motoneuron plus its axon plus the muscle fibers on which it inserts is known as the "motor unit." Approximate contraction values in gram tension were derived for motor units in different muscles. The overall picture that emerged was simple in its outlines: the fast electrical impulses (lasting 1 to 2 msec) of the input, directly or by the mediation of interneurons, bombard the synapses on the motoneuron, creating in it states of excitation or inhibition of longer duration than the impulses and capable of neutralizing each other. Somehow the net effect of $E + I$, if excitatory in character, is again transformed into impulses for the efferent motor axon. These general conclusions proved correct in principle when tested by modern micromethods of analysis, and much work has since been devoted to filling in the details as known today.

In 1929 Denny-Brown in Sherrington's laboratory succeeded in recording the electrical impulses of a single motor unit in the ankle extensor soleus (cat) at the same time as Adrian and Bronk introduced the intramuscular needle electrode and pictured them by their more convenient technique.[132] Prior to this experiment Adrian and Zotterman (1926) had functionally isolated a single sensory fiber from a stretch-sensitive end organ in a frog muscle.[132] Their work had shown that stimulus strength (degree of extension) is encoded in terms of impulse frequency in the paper referred to. Impulse activity initiated by the motoneuron also became available for study, as recordable among the muscle fibers which its axon innervated. The arrival of an era of unitary analysis of nervous activity was recognized by a Nobel Prize to Adrian and Sherrington "for their discoveries regarding the functions of neurons." In reflex work the impulse emanating from the motoneuron gradually began to replace—for a time—the isometric myogram as the chief index of neural activity. Later on, as we shall see, the myogram reentered the scene.

At the time it was generally known that a depolarization of a polarized cell membrane, recorded as a negative potential, signified increased excitability, and in 1887 W. H. Gaskell (1847–1914) had found that an opposite or positive change of potential could be led off from the sinus region of a heart inhibited to standstill by stimulation of the vagus nerve with projections found in that region.[133] Although prone to think of excitation and inhibition as two opposite processes of otherwise similar character—in line with Ewald Hering's ideas on anabolism and katabolism (mentioned in Chapter 6)—in 1932 Sherrington nevertheless hesitated to settle for a final hypothesis about their nature. When in 1934 simultaneous records of the electrical response of the retina and the impulses in the optic nerve had shown that excitation in the nerve coincided with a negative deflection and inhibition with a positive response of the retina, Sherrington commented on this finding in a letter (July 15, 1934) to me: "The opposition of *electrical* sign for E and I respectively which you find, if we cannot connect it with the chemical aspects in view of Dale's 'acetylchol' excitation . . . may prove a key to the whole mechanism of both Exc. and Inh. It seems almost inevitable, does it not, that if the mechanism, chemical or physical, of either *E* or *I* is discovered, even merely in outline (but 'principiell') that discovery must almost contain (or involve) the finding out of the other, namely I or E?"[129]

Sherrington's prophecy proved true when the intracellular microelectrode (Ling and Gerard; Nastuk and Hodgkin[129]) was employed by J. C. Eccles and his coworkers to explore single motoneurons.[28] Synaptic excitation and inhibition, as produced by appropriate reflexes, were shown to elicit opposite changes of membrane potential of the cell, *E* depolarizing it, *I* re- or hyperpolarizing. And so, thanks to the conceptual developments in reflexology, the two basic neural functional states, excitation and inhibition, had been defined in electrical units, and the field was cleared for their analysis in terms of ionic permeabilities and other electrochemical approaches. As I have expressed it elsewhere: "The present generation of experimentalists would, I believe, be willing to endorse this assessment of where Sherrington made a unique contribution to their field, and those who look backwards would also be prepared to admire the sagacity by which he went in for lines of approach that became sign-posts pointed towards the future" (p. 37).[129]

The chemical results, to which Sherrington alluded in his letter, started with Otto Loewi (1873–1961).[135] He discovered in the 1920s that stimulation of the vagus nerve of a frog heart leading to diminished contraction and final standstill was of the nature of an inhibition produced by some substance that entered the fluid pumped by the excised heart (a physiological salt solution). This fluid—a quantity of the order of a cubic centimeter—when transferred to another frog heart, caused identical effects there, only somewhat weaker. The released substance proved to be acetylcholine. Then Henry Dale (1875–1968) and his coworkers showed that a close intraarterial injection of a minute dose of acetylcholine directed toward the end plates (synapses) of the motor axons of a limb muscle excited the muscle to contract. As with the frog heart, perfusion of the muscle also set free acetylcholine into the perfusate. In 1936, Loewi and Dale shared the Nobel Prize "for their discoveries relating to chemical transmission of nerve impulses."[136] The chemistry and physiology of synaptic transmission has since been pursued in many laboratories all over the world.

The best model of synaptic transmission is still the motor end plate: the efferent motor impulses release acetylcholine, which elicits a depolarizing motor end plate potential. This in turn excites the electrochemical mechanism of the muscle fiber at a firing rate proportional to the magnitude of the end plate potential as determined by the quantity of chemical transmitter released. Every step in this act of transmission has since been analyzed in detail by Bernhard Katz and his coworkers.[137] Similarly, at the input to a neuron, the nervous impulse releases a synaptic transmitter that depolarizes the cell membrane in excitation and hyperpolarizes it in inhibition. Whether a synapse is excitatory or inhibitory depends on the nature of the subsynaptic elaboration of the structure within the piece of membrane underneath it. Much detailed knowledge about synapses and their transmitters, microchemical and electronmicroscopical, is available but cannot be reviewed here (Katz, Euler, and DeRobertis).[137]

Being interested in the management of nervous motor or sensory acts, we are concerned with explanations at a different level and thus chiefly in the constraints that the electrochemical nature of synaptic transmission imposes upon functional interpretation. The synaptic transmission takes time, about 0.5 to 1.0 msec (Lorente de Nó).[138] The effect of the transmitter upon the cell membrane is like a brief explosion, meaning that a long-lasting state of excitation or inhibition has to be maintained by continued bombardment of the cell with impulses, alternatively by the slow axoplasmic flow (mentioned in Chapter 3). As yet such a notion is entirely hypothetical. Delay circuits and reverberation of impulses (Forbes, Lorente de Nó)[139] in special loops have been invoked to explain maintained reflexes, and both ideas can be supported by anatomical evidence. It is easy enough to show, for example, that a flexor reflex is activated from many spinal segments from which the efferent impulses reach the muscle after different latent periods; hence, they are differentially delayed. Furthermore, the strategic location of the synapses, whether on the cell body or its dendrites, plays a partly understood role, and so do their different transmitter substances, the total number of which is still unknown.

It must be admitted that the need for chemically different transmitters at different synapses is not yet fully understood. Our electrical records, both intra- and extracellular, are manifestations of one particular activity, the one we actually observe and use analytically in the ways I have been discussing. It is almost a postulate that the synaptic activity some day will be shown to have some function concerned with the stamping-in of engrams, very likely by chemical markers. In this process specification by different chemical transmitters may play a role.

The decisive advance in understanding of cellular organizations, made possible by the single-cell approach, must not let us forget that animals also exhibit systemic types of control such as states of rage, voluptuousness, or sleep and wakefulness that may be held apart by large central organizations dependent on different synaptic transmitters, specific for each state. Two transmitters, acetylcholine and noradrenaline, seem to be engaged in the opposing but complementary states of sleep and wakefulness. A modern technique making use of fluorescence (Eränkö, Hillarp and Falck)[140] in staining for transmitters such as noradrenalin and serotonin has revealed systems and tracts that are homogeneous with respect to these substances. We can look forward to an era of functional identification of the systemic significance of the transmitter differentiation that has been thus disclosed.

Returning to the two best defined functional processes, excitation and inhibition, and their role in interpreting the environment and acting on it, we must emphasize that graded inhibition is the crucial modeling instrument, producing the necessary specification of action by curtailing unwanted inputs to a cell and stabilizing performance. In the latter task the negative feedback mechanism based on recurrent fibers is of fundamental importance. Without inhibition, individual cells could never have reached the high degree of specificity by overlapping excitations alone in the representation of the environment that was described in the previous chapter for visual cells of the cortex. Action is similarly specified and, in fact, the reflex arc was the first properly analyzed example of neuronal specificity of action tying, for instance, the receptors of a precise patch on the skin to a specific final common path. Between the acts most motoneurons have to be silent, and this state, too, is achieved by tonically active inhibitory projections on them that come from several supraspinal, spinal, and peripheral sources.

Another fundamental line of understanding to which we were led by reflexology concerns circuits or "wiring diagrams." To begin with, these were schematic representations of convergence and divergence on the motoneurons. But with the definite evidence (P. Hoffmann, Lloyd)[141] for a direct monosynaptic transmission of rapidly conducted impulses, soon shown to come from the primary muscle spindle afferents, one clearly defined circuit was available which began at an end organ that projected its excitatory synapses on the motoneurons of its own muscle. Branches of the same afferent fibers were found to exert an inhibitory action on the muscle's antagonist, a manifestation of the principle of reciprocal innervation. In the end, the inhibitory projections were found to be disynaptic (Eccles),[28] that is, an internuncial neuron intervenes as a kind of commutator switching the afferent synaptic effect from plus (E on this neuron) to minus I on the antagonist's motoneurons. This general type of circuit, which in this example is organized for alternating (reciprocal) flexion and extension, is one of Nature's inventions that are put to many-sided applications in the central nervous system.

Today wiring diagrams within neural centers are largely based on intracellular recording that, for identifiable cells, has provided ways to distinguish E and I synaptic potentials within a mixed output, even when for one reason or another the cell does not fire impulses.[28] In the much analyzed retina, wiring diagrams connecting its five types of neurons (receptor, bipolar, horizontal, amarcrine, and ganglion cells) have reached a degree of perfection hardly matched anywhere, excepting always a number of monosynaptic reflex arcs (Dowling and Boycott; Tomita).[142]

The reflex in Sherrington's words is a very elementary "item of behavior," but it had to be elementary to inspire the achievements that led to the understanding of synaptic action. These items of behavior still serve as useful tests in today's studies of principles of regulation. Obviously it has been recognized for a long time that spinal centers are governed by hierarchic supraspinal ones, and the term "center" is defined as an organized structure of subunits within a larger organization. Lately the shift of interest to control problems has turned up a reverse, expressing itself in a disparaging attitude toward reflexology. However, any approach to the central nervous system that can be handled with a reasonable degree of accuracy always retains its value. It is merely a question of finding new wine for the old bottles. I intend to show that this is what actually happened. The modern era of research in this field, although it is concerned with basic principles and circuits in the regulation of posture and movement, again used the reflex as a takeoff point in its reorientation of interest. In the next section I shall show what this attitude did for us and where we landed.

Afferent and Efferent Control of Tension and Extension

The stretch reflex of Liddell and Sherrington is dependent on the monosynaptic reflex arc.[35] As stated, it begins in the stretch-sensitive primary ending of the muscle spindle and excites the motoneurons of its own muscle. The reflex is supported polysynaptically; that is, by impulses from branches of the monosynaptic afferents that contact interneurons. If, for instance, the vestibular influence from the central nuclei of the balance organs is blocked, the stretch reflex loses its tonic character. As explained in Chapter 2, the response to stretch can be regarded as an example of negative feedback because lengthening (stretching) of a limb muscle is counteracted by the shortening induced by the reflex contraction of the same muscle.[132] When cybernetic science arose much later in the 1940s it was a simple example for a triumphant illustration of means of quantifying nervous processes by cybernetics[34] (see full discussion in Chapter 10).

However, falling between experimental physiology and the mathematical tool of cybernetics, Nature proved too inventive to adapt itself straightaway to the latter. Many unexpected facts were still missing that could only be discovered by patient physiological experimentation; without them the field would have become prematurely sterilized by cybernetic dogma. Further work showed that the muscle spindle, placed in parallel with the main muscle's contractile fibers and hence bound to be unloaded and silenced when the latter contracted, refused to behave in the predicted manner in "natural" activity of its muscle.[3,46] It was silenced only by artificial, electrically elicited contractions and by brief reflex tendon jerks. The decisive new factor was the evidence that the spindle is under the influence of its own separate motor fibers, the gamma fibers of Leksell.[143] These often proved to be excited (and also inhibited) in parallel with the corresponding events in the main muscle's motor fibers, the alpha fibers. Excitation of gamma motor fibers contracts the muscular poles of the spindle whose endings in the equatorial region are stretched and respond by discharging.

There are accordingly two types of motoneurons in the spinal cord: alpha motoneurons for the main muscle and gamma motoneurons for the muscular apparatus of the spindles, its intrafusal muscle fibers. Thus the gamma motoneurons operate a loop through the spindles back to the spinal cord (Figure 7.1). In most natural motor acts that have been studied, the two systems, alpha and gamma, appear to be closely linked in action. The neural mechanism of this alpha-gamma linkage is not everywhere known in detail, but its effect, coexcitation or coinhibition, has been extensively studied. In coexcitation the intrafusal muscle is contracted together with the (main) extrafusal partner, so the ending can fire throughout the contractile response behaving outwardly almost as a tendon organ recording tension. An electrically elicited muscle twitch, stimulating only alpha fibers, immediately induces a pause in the discharge because the spindle—in parallel with the main muscle—is being briefly unloaded. By this test the tendon organ—in series with the main muscle—would record increased tension. With coinhibition the spindle is slackened together with the main muscle, hence lengthened without producing a discharge to lengthening (stretch). The essential spindle problems were thus shifted from a simple application of feedback theory to the highly complex questions of how and why the gamma-spindle

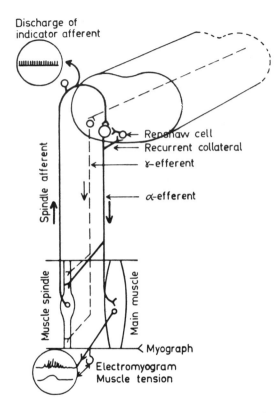

7.1. Diagram of extrafusal and intrafusal innervation of muscle and the circuits involved. The muscle spindle with its large primary afferent placed in parallel with the main muscle, sends its message monosynaptically to the motoneurons in the spinal cord. The ventral horn cell is provided with a recurrent collateral through the Renshaw cell. The gamma motor nerves (broken line) lead to the muscular poles of the spindle which they contract, thereby exerting a pull on the sense organ. The supraspinal control of the gamma motoneurons is indicated (within the spinal cord). For analysis, this circuit can be intercepted at several points but the diagram shows only a recording from a branch of the dorsal root as well as a myogram and electromyogram. All results are displayed on cathode ray oscillographs.

loop performs its regulatory functions, whatever they be.[37] Some details are required for understanding these relationships which deliver paradigmatic illustrations of how the nervous apparatus handles control problems, motor to be sure, but at the same time with general applicability. My description will be based on the spindle's primary end organ. Its other, secondary end organ will be briefly mentioned.

Both endings are placed in the equatorial middle between two muscular poles and the whole spindlelike organ lies between the extrafusal or main muscle fibers in parallel with them. If the spindle's intrafusal muscles are excited by gamma impulses, the ensuing contraction stretches the equatorial endings; the greater their tension, the higher their firing rate. A tense spindle is also more sensitive to brief phasic stretches, testable by vibratory stimulation. It follows higher frequencies of the vibrator. It may or may not have become more sensitive in absolute terms; that is, the slope of the curve relating its impulse frequency to degree of stretching may or may not have become steeper; at any rate, it is within the means of the gamma motor fibers to produce also a great increase of sensitivity in the spindle endings.[46]

After reading Chapter 6, it should be evident that no sense organ is designed for meaningless operations. When the clinician pulls on the muscles of a normal subject, the stretch reflex effect is negligible. This act is biologically meaningless for an end organ that is supposed to work in relation to linked commands arriving in parallel to both alpha and gamma motoneurons. In man, strong maintained stretch reflexes are a pathological sign to be interpreted as a pure excitatory surplus from some source, but perhaps more often as a release of the alpha motoneurons from necessary tonic inhibitions with hyperexcitability as its net effect.[37] A release of the gamma motoneurons or, alternatively, an excitatory process keeping them hyperactive, would also lead to exaggerated stretch reflexes by virtue of the properties of the gamma-spindle loop. The best example experimenters have found of hyperactive gamma motoneurons is the stretch reflex of the decerebrated rigid animal. The stretch reflex was originally discovered in this preparation. In Parkinson's disease, a rigid state with exaggerated stretch reflexes as a prominent symptom, there is actually a heightened level of spindle activity (Hagbarth), demonstrable by direct recording from the nerve by the technique of Hagbarth and Vallbo.[144] This discharge must be caused by gamma fiber hyperactivity resulting from either of the two reasons given.

The absence of alpha motor activity in sleep and drowsiness is also characterized by low activity in the gamma system and hence by slow or absent spontaneous firing on the part of the muscle spindles. As soon as an animal is alerted to arousal, it automatically throws its gamma system into action. The ensuing increased spindle activity raises the level of excitability of the alpha motoneurons across the gamma loop and must also contribute to inducing a state of preparedness in supraspinal centers such as the cerebral cortex and the cerebellum onto which spindle afferents project.[46] One visible effect is a general increase of tone.

More often the term "tone" or "tonus" is used as a synonym for postural reflexes, that is, for readjustments to gravity. Before there was any experimental material in this field, Rossi (1927) had suggested that the central nervous system had entrusted the maintenance and initiation of postural adjustments to what much later became known as the gamma loop across the spindles.[145] This idea presupposes that spindle activity should precede alpha motor activity and, as a matter of fact, in these slow reflexes it often does. Thus, when the gamma-sensitized spindle is stretched under the influence of gravity, the ensuing stretch reflex can compensate for this effect. The alpha motoneuron is in this way relieved of maintaining a permanent low-grade activity to preserve an equally permanent readiness to check minor variations of loading. It is all handled automatically by the reflex from the sensitized length-detector throwing in its alpha partner only when a correction of muscle length is required, a most economical arrangement. This is only one role ascribed to the gamma loop.

A considerable body of evidence shows that the gamma loop plays a decisive role in postural adjustments. In the laboratory animals these reflexes are operated by special motor units (see Chapter 2) collected in slow, "red" bundles of muscle fibers capable of the sustained tonic contractions needed in adjustments to gravity. In the cat the motoneurons of these muscles are provided with a denser network of projections from primary spindle endings than the fast and powerful "white" muscles. They are thus sensitive to activation across the gamma loop.[37]

Muscles that are richly provided with spindles tend to be the ones that do not undergo great physiological changes of length in contraction, such as neck muscles, the deep red portions of limb muscles, adductors and abductors of the limbs, and the small muscles of the finger tips. Meticulous length control or maintenance of a precise length setting is the purpose served by an abundant supply of these length detectors. One need only think of localization by hearing

or sight to realize the need for a fixed position of the head
or, for that matter, of the skill displayed by Oriental wom-
en in carrying water jars on their heads.
With the stretch reflex goes load compensation, directly
demonstrated for certain muscles, for example, in respiration (C. v. Euler; Sears).[146] For this the spindles must be
activated, either tonically or coactivated in alpha-gamma
linkage. An unexpected load stretches a muscle whose
spindles respond by facilitating a contraction to resist the
change. Sudden unloading leads to the opposite effect: the
muscle shortens, thus silencing its spindles which become
too long relative to the length of the main muscle. This
temporarily relieves the motoneuron of excitation. Thus,
like a thermoregulatory device consisting of a sensor and
an energy source, the spindle contributes to maintaining a
desired degree of contraction. The spindle is the sensor
and the motor unit the energy source in this natural servomechanism. But although the sensor of a thermoregulator
is adjusted for one particular temperature, the gamma-
controlled spindle is adjustable for any desired length setting and in addition adjustable in sensitivity. How and
when a freely moving subject makes use of this exquisite
control circuit is still something of a question. Only a limited choice of situations is available to the experimenter.
    For maintaining a length setting, it is important that the
sensitivity of the primary ending in impulses per millimeter of extension has been found to be highest for small
stretches. Also the gamma motoneurons are separable into
two types: one is dynamic, increasing the output from the
spindle during the actual process of stretching, the more
so, the greater the velocity of stretch; the other is static,
keeping up spindle activity in maintained contractions
(Matthews).[147] Like many other end organs, the muscle

spindle is sensitive to rate of stimulation (rate of stretching), and this property is controlled by the dynamic gamma fibers. In servotheory terms this means that the immediate rise in firing rate by derivative feedback compensates for the delay between the response of the sensor and the muscular act. This transport lag across the reflex arc tends to place the contraction of the muscle so much out of phase with the preceding signal to contract that the circuit, without the spindle's rate sensitivity, might go into oscillations.

I have taken up these facts and ideas, many of which have been derived from work with the stretch reflex, in some detail because they illustrate the applicability of general regulation science to a particular circuit with a partly known wiring diagram. They do establish for nervous circuits the validity of principles of control applied in the numerous servomechanisms with electrical and mechanical components that surround our daily life. Having admitted as much, I must—in justice to Nature's inventiveness—also point out that we have only looked at one particular aspect of gamma-spindle control. The other end organ within the muscle spindle, its secondary ending, has different reflex actions in flexors and extensors, and the static gamma fibers excite both primary and secondary endings together. The dynamic ones are restricted in their action to the primary end organ that I have discussed (Barker; Boyd; Laporte).[148] And when considering muscular afferents, it is at least necessary to include also the tendon organs that record tension. In muscular acts both extension and tension are under control by end organs, which have their regulatory mechanisms within the spinal cord. Tendon organs, wherever found, have inhibitory actions on motoneurons of their own muscles. A purposive choice by the motor organization determines whether this inhibition shall be on or off. And so the attractive, basic simplicity of servocircuitry turns out to be loaded with complications: there are three overlapping reflexes to stretch instead of only one because all three end organs are stretch-sensitive in their own different ways. Two are controlled by motor fibers inside the muscle and the third (from the tendon organ) largely by supraspinal fibers descending to the spinal cord. Experimenters can go a long way on servotheory with each of them individually. They can define boundary conditions for their operations, but they have not yet succeeded in doing what a brain does automatically with the greatest ease whenever it evaluates their joint action and adjusts each of them for an optimal share within a total act in relation to simultaneous information from joint and skin receptors around them—the whole act being in addition supervised or even initiated by the eyes.

As stated previously, the muscular end organs also project to the cerebral cortex and to the cerebellum. Many cortical and cerebellar sites are engaged in controlling spindle sensitivity, to judge by the experimental finding that virtually every cortical, cerebellar, or subcortical structure from which the alpha motoneurons can be influenced likewise influences the discharge from the gamma motoneurons.[46] Their activity, of course, is reflected in the rate of firing of the muscle spindles. Voluntary movement in hand muscles has been studied by recording with microelectrodes from single spindle afferents in human subjects. These experiments showed that there was spindle coactivation in the small, relatively fast and homogeneous muscles concerned (Hagbarth and Vallbo). Although the gamma path is slower than the alpha path and its effect is delayed in the spindle loop, nevertheless it proved fast enough in these experiments to produce spindle coactivation on the rising phase of the recorded contractions, even when they were very brief.

Because the voluntary contraction is of complex origin and expresses a demand, it must be concluded that spindle coactivation signifies that the same demand is also represented by instructions to the gamma motoneurons. It is difficult to conceive of any other role for this duplication of voluntary commands than that the spindles are coactivated also to feed back information on whether the motor act actually accomplished the demanded result. In the event of a failure, the peripheral loop would produce whatever correction is in its power, as explained previously, and inform the central structures about it. Other sense organs such as the eyes and those in joints and skin contribute to feedback in aid of error correction, but only the muscular endings are directly concerned with the performance of the muscles in terms of their own parameters of function. Spindles are, as it were, private sensors for the muscles.

My emphasis on alpha-gamma linkage and thus on coactivation does not imply that alpha and gamma neurons could not act independently. If linked action were the only mode of function, then evolution of the mammalian gamma-spindle apparatus would never have occurred, because in the frog the muscle spindles are innervated solely by branches of the alpha fibers and thus automatically coactivated by this peripheral mechanism. Mammals have only a few alpha branches peripheral to spindles. Encephalization, here as in so many other cases, has favored individualization and independence by developing alpha and gamma motoneurons and linking them centrally when coexcitation or coinhibition is purposive for a motor act. My emphasis on alpha-gamma linkage is motivated by the fact that this state of affairs is a common experimental finding. Independent action of the two types of motoneurons can be used purposively in correspondence to appropriate needs, but is not always so easy to imitate experimentally. I have been discussing automatic processes, but do the muscle spindles and tendon organs in addition give rise to any specific percepts? My general standpoint is the same as in the previous chapter—if any sensible need arises for perceiving any afferent message to the cortex, it will be perceived. Both old and new evidence favors a perception of graded resistance or force from muscular afferents, but the main concern of the supraspinal stations is to automatize movement control as soon as possible rather than to keep it going at the level of full awareness. Movements that begin under visual control tend to develop by practice in the direction of pure proprioceptive and skin control. Recent information shows skin afferents to be very important. They are, for instance, needed for acquiring control over a prosthesis (Moberg).[56]

8
Current Ideas on
Brain Control of Movement

The cerebral cortex is responsible for goal-directed behaviour. (D. Denny-Brown, *The Cerebral Control of Movement*. Liverpool University Press, 1966, p. 199.)

Hierarchic Subdivision of Control

From the last century has come down to us the question of whether the brain operates in terms of muscles or movements (Hughlings Jackson).[4] Phillips, siding with Hughlings Jackson, the distinguished nineteenth-century neurologist, quotes him: "There are, we shall say, thirty muscles of the hand; these are represented in the nervous centers in thousands of different combinations—that is, as very many movements; it is just as many chords, musical expressions and tunes can be made out of a few 'notes'."[149] Clearly the regulated quantity is movement but, if our goal is to move a single muscle, this—in some cases—can be done. As students of the organization of movement we are interested in the "intracerebral selector mechanisms which can activate and inhibit the 'points de depart' in 'thousands of different combinations'" (Phillips). This amounts to realizing that we must endeavor to analyze them at different hierarchic levels, beginning at the motor unit and ending with the cortex and its goal-directed behavior.

The introductory quotation may look like a truism, considering that purposiveness prevails everywhere in the nervous system, but it was chosen to emphasize that encephalization has left the cortex in supreme control of purpose. In men and monkeys the cortex is possessed of every bit of the information that is needed for posture and movement, including knowledge of how muscles insert, whether across one joint or two, what motor units they contain, and many other boundary conditions.

The motor units represent an array of different properties—slow, fast, phasic, tonic, weak, powerful—all of which answer definite needs that in turn are caused by the tasks allotted to individual muscles. In some muscles, the motor units are highly differentiated; in others, fairly homogeneous. Of the latter type are, for instance, the slow ones in the calf-extensor soleus. As an example of a highly differentiated muscle I shall take the cat's medial gastrocnemius, one of the four extensor muscles that jointly form the tendon of Achilles at the heel. The other three are the lateral gastrocnemius, the plantaris, and the soleus. The medial gastrocnemius has been studied in great detail, and my choice is motivated for both this reason and because it shows how insertion of several muscles at the same tendon does not prevent them from subserving different functions.[150] This illustrates that at the lowest level of nervous hierarchic control, the element controlled is the motor unit.

The slow units of the gastrocnemius muscle are as slow as those of the soleus. They tend to be red, to have little power but much endurance, and to be run by small tonic motoneurons of slow-conduction velocity. At the other end of the spectrum are the fast and powerful "white" units innervated by rapidly conducting motor axons of large motoneurons engaged in phasic activities. In between are some units of intermediate properties. Long ago it was noticed by Denny-Brown that the soleus was inhibited to stimulation of the motor cortex while the gastrocnemius was excited.[151] Thus the tonic soleus, important for postural adjustments to gravity, was eliminated when the powerful gastrocnemius took over, possibly a combination realized in stepping. At that time experiments were not yet carried out in terms of motor units, and so it was not known what the slow units of gastrocnemius might have done during the presumed step.

Complete information can be obtained by intracellular recording and stimulation from the tip of the inserted microelectrode.[150] When this was done, the important parameter in heterogeneous muscles like gastrocnemius proved to be the motor unit and not the whole muscle as such. Thus, for instance, the synaptic organization is different for the slow and the fast units of gastrocnemius; there is more disynaptic inhibition from an antagonist flexor and also more monosynaptic excitation from muscle spindle afferents on the slow than on the fast motor units. Descending tracts also treat slow and fast units differently. The slow fatigue-resistant muscle fibers of tonic motoneurons support the sustained stretch reflex, which, as we know, is subject to central control, not only by the gamma system but also from the nuclei on to which fibers from the balance organs in the ear project.[37]

Movements can never be discussed as if they took place in a vacuum. An internal representation of the external world is available at the hierarchic top level and the brain is cognizant of it in planning any motor act (Chapter 9). Sherrington emphasized the role of the "distance receptors" as a unifying influence from the cerebral hemispheres contributing to the "solidarity of the motor creature" by integrating long series of reactions of the animal as a whole. In programming a movement, we are not aware of choosing the required amount of alpha-gamma linkage and the correct subcortical routes. We simply demand an end result—often visualized—and check it by impulses fed back from muscles, joints, skin, and eyes. The "demand" injects purpose into the motor act. As to the rest, we rely on the organization, partly laid down genetically, partly by experience, and expect it to obey its own rules of the game. This organization is perfect enough in monkeys to function in the absence of its cortical pyramidal components.

Nothing prevents us from thinking in terms of single

muscles, if this is what we demand. A large number of muscles can be contracted individually. Others can only be actuated together in established combinations and sequences. Swallowing is a sequential action run on each side by twelve muscles. It can be reflexively triggered into activity but not subdivided (Doty).[152] Opening the fist for a handshake requires activation of a large number of small hand and wrist muscles in precisely gated, successive entries (Duchenne).[153] Few, if any, can be excited individually. At the other end of the scale it is nevertheless possible for us to activate voluntarily even single motor units, at least of some muscles. Success presupposes that a reliable feedback is established by leading the electrical impulse of a motor unit to the screen of an oscillograph to be seen or to a loudspeaker so that it can be heard. By such "knowledge of result" as a guide we can adjust the amount of our volitional effort until the response seen or heard consists of a single impulse (Basmajian).[154]

Thus, for the cortex, the decisive question is the purpose of the movement, whether to walk, to type, to pick up a raisin, or to play with a single motor unit. Experimenters, on their side, want to know how motor control is organized at the different hierarchic levels. The finally relevant conclusion is drawn by the motor unit, which represents direct access to the forces, its own internal as well as external ones.

Internuncial Bias

The word "bias" is a metaphor borrowed by physiology from the original triode valve of the early amplifiers. The grid between the anode and the cathode of the vacuum tube is given a "grid bias" of potential that determines the amount of current flowing through the tube. A small

change of grid bias causes a large change of current and thus controls the amount of amplification.

Assume that a motoneuron at a membrane potential of -70 mv needs to be at -55 mv to be able to discharge. There are a number of excitatory biasing mechanisms in addition to tonic firing from monosynaptic afferents. They are carried by internuncial cells (interneurons), which are actuated by spinal reflexes and by supraspinal descending pathways. Afferent nerve impulses from sense organs combine at interneuronal cells with supraspinal descending impulses in processes of interaction to form purposive patterns for exciting or inhibiting motoneurons. By counteracting the tonic inhibitory bias, synapses from interneurons may keep a motoneuron at a membrane potential close to its firing level so that a small additional depolarization suffices to make it spill over into discharging. Rarely if ever does a motoneuron fire to one isolated excitatory input. But the internuncial apparatus does what the gamma motor fibers do for the muscle spindle by contracting their intrafusal fibers; it determines the motoneuron's bias from moment to moment, as required by the task in hand. Across the gamma loop through the spindles the motoneurons in addition are gamma-biased.

As the internuncial cells are structurally organized or wired up, they represent purposive combinations of various supraspinal, intraspinal, and peripheral influences (Sherrington).[96] Thus, for instance, internuncial cells A may represent a combination of motoneurons in muscles x, y, and z, while the internuncials B put the motoneurons to work in connection with those of muscles p, u, and v, perhaps at the same time inhibiting motoneurons in muscles x, y, and z. Quite complex organizations of this type may be wholly spinal and merely controlled by supraspinal centers as elucidated by Lundberg and his group in Gothenburg.[155]

For example, if a spinal cat is lifted up from the neck, the hanging hind limbs start walking, at any rate if one leg is pulled to initiate the act. This means that the basic organization for walking is localized in the spinal cord. It is supported by the reciprocally organized reflexes from the limb muscles. Flexors and extensors around the same joint are kept to alternate action by reciprocal innervation. But even in the absence of this input from the limb, the animal may walk. We can think of this example as a model of a triggered movement. The rhythmic organization in the spinal cord merely needs a push to get started. Stimulation of the midbrain, in the absence of the rest of the brain, is all that is needed to initiate and maintain stepping in the cat (Severin, Shik, and Orlovskij).[156] The midbrain must contain a number of "command" neurons capable of activating the spinal gait mechanism.

This concept, command neuron, has turned up in the studies of invertebrate rhythmic movements (Wiersma; Kennedy and Davis).[157] In crustaceans each of a few identifiable internuncial neurons is capable of starting a rhythmic movement of the swimming foot of the lobster. The individual command neurons do not have exactly the same output and none can elicit the full range of movement in locomotion that a few can produce by summation. The essential point, however, is that the act is organized as a fixed program run by a few push buttons. In addition the running program—as in mammals—is modifiable by sensory feedback. The muscular sense organs in some invertebrates are also controlled by motor fibers.

Though the number of command neurons is so small in the lobster that they can be counted, the same limitation need not hold for man or monkey. A decisive factor must be the degree of adaptability and complexity of the repertoire of movements of an organism. The cyclic oscillation of the swimming foot of a crustacean is simple compared with what the human hand has to accomplish. However, the existence of command neurons underlines the validity of a principle of economy, an ideal minimum of mobilizers of effort. Something like this recurs in the finding of electroencephalographers that large portions of the cortex are activated while a dog is being trained to execute a conditioned reflex. When activation ultimately is well established, the cortical activity turns out to be restricted to one specific site. Generalizing from these experiences, it seems reasonable to expect the number of command neurons needed for initiating a cyclic movement like walking, or a well-fixated automatism like swallowing, to be small compared with the number required for the numerous voluntary movements of the hand. For mammals it is not possible to mention any figures, as shown in the next section.

Voluntary Movement

If purposiveness more obviously lies on the surface in the motor than in the sensory field, so does anticipation. Independently of whether an act is voluntary or automatic, laid down in the genome or developed under full conscious awareness, it presupposes anticipation of a goal. In voluntary motor acts electronic summation of the events at a number of electrodes on the scalp can be used to obtain some insight into the ongoings of the cortex. Man and monkey have served in such experiments in many laboratories. They show that complex changes of electrical potential precede the final contraction of the muscles to be activated. Beginning some 800 msec before this moment, there is a bilateral, drawn out, not specifically localized cortical process, the readiness potential (Kornhuber and Deecke).[158] About 50 to 150 msec before contraction, a more precise and brisk motor potential is observed over the part of the motor area belonging to the muscles called up for service.

Compared with the findings presented here, this information may seem to be meager, but it does show (1) that an important part of the voluntary act is processed in the cortex as a spatiotemporal pattern, (2) that the demand for action uses a very large number of cells in many different cortical sites, (3) that demanding within the cortex lasts a long time compared with the speed of the impulse over the short distances in it, and (4) that in the end a motor command is focused on the motor area.

During this drawn-out processing of the voluntary movement, the cortex has had time to explore a large amount of stored and incoming information from skin, joints, muscles, and balance organs. These senses have projections that are adjacent to those of the motor area. Advance information is highly relevant, relating to the initial position of the limb that is supposed to execute the demanded act. By preventing information from the limb from reaching the brain, it is possible to obtain an idea of whether such information meant anything for the cortical processing of the motor act. Such experiments have been done (Vaughan, Gross, and Bossom),[159] and they show that without impulses from the limb the motor potential still appears and in gross outline is similar to its normal version but is now much retarded and prolonged. It may be twice as late and twice as long.

The finding implies that during processing of a demanded act the cortex takes in and uses information from limb afferents in elaborating a wanted movement. At the level of encephalization of a monkey, the motor cortex must be cognizant of the peripheral conditions for the movement: for example, where in space the limb happens to be, what muscles are in operation and to what extent they are engaged, and which ones are inhibited. Without such information the demanded movement can take place, but it is delayed and has lost in precision of execution.

In current discussions of preprogramming versus continuous modeling and phasing of a motor act by sensory feedback from the periphery, those favoring the former alternative have been able to refer to much experimental evidence showing that the essential patterning of a movement is retained after exclusion of peripheral afferent information. The experiment on motor potentials in the absence of peripheral information confirms the existence of a cortical program. At the same time it shows that for speed and precision preprogramming requires some basic information from the periphery. But many stereotyped or very fast motor acts may well be wholly preprogrammed in the cortex the way reflexes are programmed in the spinal cord. My own view is that nothing can be gained by polarizing this problem around two mutually exclusive alternatives. When we know—as we do today—that in man the voluntary commands in many movements are distributed to both alpha and gamma motoneurons (Hagbarth and Vallbo)[144] and that the latter activate the muscle spindles, then common sense indicates the conclusion that the elaborate gamma-spindle apparatus, ending up with cortical projections, hardly can be irrelevant for the act in which it participates. The demand, expressed in alpha-gamma coactivation, is likely to require the spindles for checking accomplishment.

It should be realized, too, that preparation of a voluntary movement extends far down into the spinal cord and even engages muscles that do not have a share in it. This conclusion has been reached by monosynaptic testing of the level of excitability of the alpha motoneurons. A weak electrical shock is applied to the large and fast spindle afferent fibers. In man these are accessible at some point where the nerve fibers run close to the surface (Hoffmann).[141] The shock elicits a small monosynaptic reflex from the motoneurons. The response can be recorded from the motor units in the tested muscle. Assume that a voluntary movement is assigned to the right soleus while the left soleus is ordered to remain in the resting state. The experiment begins with a warning signal, followed by a preparatory period ending with the signal to act. During the preparatory period the excitability rises in the motoneuron pools of both the right and the left soleus, which is proved by the bilaterally increased size of the monosynaptic reflex.

This experiment (Requin and Paillard)[160] has been modified in many ways, and both inhibition and excitation by the monosynaptic index can be seen to be involved in the preparatory adjustments of resting and active muscles. The muscles not engaged in the demanded movement appear to be held in readiness, as it were, on the chance that the planned movement might develop into one or another of several possible directions suggested by experience and laid down in the spinal cord. Such "ghost" movements seem to be part of the purposive strategy of the conscious brain. They are in themselves subconscious, but if the nature of the demand is varied, they too vary in a sensible manner.

All this suggests that such early "ghost" movements at least partly originate in the motor area, which has monosynaptic projections on the alpha executive in the spinal cord (Bernhard and Bohm)[161] and some also on the gamma motoneurons (Phillips).[161] Most projections from the motor area are, however, polysynaptic and act—as stated—on the interneurons in the ventral horn of the spinal cord. These, in close proximity to the motoneurons, are organized as a kind of substructure for the facilitation of several standard motor acts. A fraction of the total order is reflected as "ghost" movements. The cortex thus operates definite spinal cord sets or, in the words of Denny-Brown (1966): "The patterns of activity of the spinal organization predetermine the patterns of pyramidal activation and selection" (p.207).[162] (The pyramids descend from the motor area to the spinal cord.)

The Pyramidal Tract and the Motor Area

Most studies of the pyramidal tract (pathway) deal with the fibers that originate in the motor area and end in the spinal cord. One reason for the special interest in this cortical region is that it has been known for a hundred years (Fritsch and Hitzig, 1870)[163] as an electrically excitable area producing motor effects, another reason that early histology was good enough to demonstrate that the fibers concerned traveled in the pyramids—elongated pyramidiform structures visible from the outside below a brain turned upside down. The pyramidal output is largely crossed so that left and right motor areas excite muscles on opposite sides of the body.

Movements are also governed by the cerebellum and by subcortical centers. There is at least one supplementary motor area, but only the pyramidal tract is well enough analyzed to illustrate a few basic organizational rules. Upward in the phylum the pyramidal system has expanded in size to a maximum fiber content of about 1 million in man. The teleological asset favoring this expansion is held to have been the development of the hand from a general "power grip" to the "precision grip" of thumb and index (Phillips).[16] This also tells us something about pyramidal function. The important extrapyramidal mechanisms of motor control, as such well established, require anatomy at a level far beyond what is feasible here.

Our ideas on the nature of pyramidal control of move- ment are derived from three main sources: detailed histology, microphysiological analytical work, and such op- erative techniques as section of the pyramids or ablation of the cortical motor area, followed by studies of behavioral deficits. Additional information comes from the clinic. His- tology and microphysiology cooperate in searching out analytical elements on which to build up understanding in terms of cell types, synaptic arrangements, and wiring dia- grams with functional implications. The clinician has less use for this variety of insight; he is more interested in the effects of section and ablation on behavior, which can be compared with pathological anatomy and clinical symp- toms of damage or destruction of identifiable regions of the brain. In the end the clinical and theoretical approaches must come together by converging toward complementary explanations. A major obstacle is that the experimental experience ends at the level of the monkey whereas pyramidal control is stepped up some degrees in the design of the brain of man.

The pyramidal tract is not exclusive for the motor area. Its origin is more extensive, including parts of the parietal brain (Figures 4.3 and 4.4) and the "postcentral" sites belonging to the somatic sensory area lying behind the central sulcus that may be said to divide the brain into an anterior motor and a posterior sensory half. The cells of origin of the pyramidal tract receive a sensory input whose latent period is brief in the postcentral (sensory) neurons and twice as long in precentral (motor) ones. The latter, in the motor area, thus receive it less directly. However, the motor area is kept well informed about sensory events. It has a polysensory input, meaning one from many sense organs (Albe-Fessard and Liebeskind; Buser and Imbert),[164] and much of it arrives across nuclei of the thalamus below the cortex, a major center for motor and sensory interaction.

The fibers from the postcentral cortex in the descending pyramidal tract contact sensory neurons on their way down to the spinal cord. Thus there are projections to the reticular formation, an area at the base of the brain receiving a polysensory inflow; other fibers find their way to the nuclei (at the level of the neck) of the dorsal columns, which are large spinal tracts carrying information on sensations of touch, position, and movement of the limbs. In the spinal cord the destination is the internuncial network of neurons in the region where the afferent impulses from the periphery enter the cord.

Why these particular pyramidal fibers engage sensory neurons in so many different places is known only in broad outlines. They exercise some kind of restraining influence from the cortex on the sensory input. It can be motivated by an obvious need for curtailment of this inflow. The individual sensory endings are incredibly sensitive, which sometimes is a real asset but may easily develop into a dangerous claim for monopoly of a cortex that is devoted to work at the top level of "artfulness." Its subtle operations are unlikely to be compatible with the existence of an unbridled, massive barrage of impulses from the periphery. It may be that the pyramidal path also has an important specific role of selecting the momentarily useful sensory message and suppressing the rest, but, as I said, these sensory aspects of pyramidal control have not attracted as much interest as the more obvious muscular acts, which after all represent an interpretation in themselves.

Some aspects of pyramidal motor control were mentioned in discussing processing of voluntary movement and its electrical accompaniments in the cortex and the spinal cord. As if this should not suffice to illustrate the formidable intricacy of the problem, there is the additional complication that on their way to the appropriate spinal segments the descending pyramidal fibers dispatch collateral branches to many of the subcortical sites, which produce organized movements on stimulation, as well as to the cerebellum. The same sites dispatch fibers to the motor cortex.

What can we understand of such an incredibly complex information and command system? There is a limit to the degree of ignorance permitted in the scientific use of such terms as "information" and "control." It is also unsatisfactory to regard the whole mechanism merely as a "black box" delivering an output to an input, such as a demand for a specific motor act. The temptation to give up altogether is strong when one realizes with Harmon that if one has n subsystems, the number of parameters may be still larger, but even if they were n only, there would be 2^n subsets making "complete assessment . . . virtually impossible if n is large" (p. 488).[165] My personal reply to this is that scientists may have to abandon the hope of ever understanding the whole miraculous performance of our sensorimotor brain, but they can never give up searching for leading principles of organization.

By briefly reviewing two types of experiments, I shall try to illustrate the kinds of explanations that modern microelectrode techniques have made possible. One of them (Phillips)[161] dealt with selective surface stimulation of a group of the large cortical neurons called Betz cells after their discoverer (1874). The effect of the stimulus was recorded by intracellular microelectrodes within the motoneurons to which a group of Betz cells, a so-called colony, had access. The recorded response was a monosynaptic membrane potential of the motoneuron in the spinal cord.

As the stimulating cortical electrode was shifted across a colony without change of stimulus strength, a best point was found at which the response of the impaled motoneuron was maximal. Outside the best point, the size of the response diminished toward the edge of the colony. The colonies were found to overlap in distribution, which apparently signifies that the impaled motoneuron takes part in different functional combinations of muscles. The large thumb area in Figure 4.5 shows that thumb movements have many degrees of freedom. Very narrow colonies with high response maxima of their motoneurons were characteristic of the distal hand muscles; upward along the limb the cortical area of each colony expanded while the monosynaptic response of its motoneuron diminished. Control of the small hand muscles is thus both stronger and more precisely specified than it is for limb muscles.

Stimulation of a colony only elicited a depolarizing monosynaptic potential of its motoneuron but did not fire it unless the motoneuron was biased from some other source. Repetition of the cortical stimulus led to a cumulative increase of the postsynaptic depolarizing potential. One important source of bias was soon discovered. It turned out that the motoneurons with strong monosynaptic projections from the cortex (distal hand muscles) also received powerful monosynaptic projections from the spindles in the muscles they activated. The distal hand muscles are richly provided with spindles, so a system was discovered for precise, fast cooperation between them and the motor cortex. The pyramidal monosynaptic path from the Betz cells is the fastest cortical motor route, and at the peripheral end the large monosynaptic spindle afferents with conduction velocities of maximally 120 m/sec are likewise faster than any other afferent fibers.

One can think of many uses for a fast and direct corticospinal control mechanism provided with a fast feedback. It would, for instance, be extremely valuable for rapid error correction in load compensation of motor acts involving complex delicate manipulations of small objects. The important claims of maintenance and force of a muscular effort are better satisfied by the pyramidal polysynaptic circuits, mentioned in the previous section. Such circuits also originate in the large Betz cells, which represent but a small fraction of the total pyramidal output, however, something of the order of 10 percent. Smaller cells in the motor area stand for the major part of the pyramidal tract. All complex motor acts are likely to require internuncial, that is, polysynaptically elaborated wiring diagrams at several levels in the paths descending to the spinal internuncial apparatus.

The recording of impulse activity from single sensory cells in the cortex, mentioned in Chapter 6, has its pendant in Evarts's studies of single pyramidal neurons in a monkey previously trained to flex its wrist against a variable load while rewarded for performance.[166] Both flexor and extensor pyramidal tract neurons were discovered, and the discharge rates of the cells were found to be related to force and rate of change of force, not to the degree or direction of displacement required for the task, which itself must have been ordered from a higher hierarchic level. The neuron in the motor area translated the demand into the language in which motoneurons speak to their muscles. Sometimes paired cells were located by the same external microelectrode, and these could operate both simultaneously or reciprocally, as one might have predicted from the overlap of colonies. There were also tonic pyramidal tract neurons which did not take part in the phasic wrist movements. It was noted that such neurons exert an inhibitory effect on limb extensors.

Because microelectrodes permit precise timing, it could be shown that the pyramidal instructions preceded the electromyographic response of the contracting muscles. When the wrist flexion encountered a sudden resistance and speed of action was rewarded, the pyramidal cells were informed about this resistance within 25 msec and returned an order for a stronger contraction of the muscle in load compensation within a total time of 35 msec. These times are so brief that they require the fast monosynaptic mechanism previously described.

Animals could move long before the phylogenetic appearance of the massive pyramidal tract of the primates. Ablation of the motor area or section of the pyramids in the primates confirms this, because it has been necessary to develop special, delicate tests to detect the ensuing deficiencies that, according to Denny-Brown (1966),[162] concern the precise adaptation of the movements to the spatial attributes of the stimulus. Independent activity of the index finger and the precision grip of thumb and index are other examples of acts that require an intact pyramidal tract (Phillips).[161] Evarts's technique confirms that many sites other than the motor area are engaged in the control of movement. The thalamus (the large structure below the cortex), the cerebellum, and some basal ganglia share with the motor cortex the property of firing in advance of the electromyogram of the performing muscles. Without anatomy beyond the means of this book, it is impossible to go further in discussing the significance of the widely separated structures engaged in motor control. Why so many places should be required for motor acts is a major riddle, so far unsolved. Phillips points out that "the act of grasping an object in the field of vision may start from many different postures and may reach it by as many different trajectories as there are occasions to grasp" (Hughlings Jackson Lecture).[149] This throws some light on the need for many control stations. It is also possible that controls of velocity and of balance between posture and movement are localized to specific noncortical sites of their own (Chapter 9). A major role in programming for a motor act must be ascribed to the basal ganglia of the brain and to the cerebellum, to judge by the symptoms caused by disease in these structures. The deficits observed concern essential qualities of voluntary and automatic movement such as speed, smoothness, amplitude, and power. The rest of the cortex is more likely to stand for sophistication in relation to the environment and the motor area for a command to the motoneurons (Chapter 9).

Concluding Remarks

What is volitional in a voluntary movement is its purpose.

This is put through an automatic control system of which experimenters have been able to elucidate a number of major facts and some operative principles. I refer to the selection of material presented in this and the preceding chapter: the gamma loop and alpha-gamma linkage, the specification of motor unit properties, the cortical readiness and motor potentials, the colony concept, the ghost movements, and the recording from single cortical and other neurons during intentional wrist movements. The list—by no means complete—represents an impressive number of disclosures won by dint of hard work in the laboratory. And yet the full logic of the automatic control system still eludes us. What, for instance, is the motor role of the cerebellum whose intricate wiring diagrams are quite well known (Eccles, Ito, Szenthágothai)?[167] The answer to this question is that we merely possess a number of hypotheses demonstrating that wiring diagrams have to be infused with a modicum of teleological relevance to be more than an enumeration of inhibitions and excitations at synaptic loci. Five hypotheses are mentioned by Llinás in a recent review.[168]

9
Motor and Sensory Organizations in Integrated Action

In "sensorimotor processes" in general, localization might tend to a greater degree of minuteness on the receptor than on the effector side. There must be no ambiguity about the localization of an object in the field of vision. But the part used to grasp it may start from many different postures and may reach it by as many trajectories as there are occasions to grasp. (C. G. Phillips, Cortical localization and "sensorimotor processes" at the "middle level" in primates. Hughlings Jackson Lecture, *Proc. Roy. Soc. Med.* 66 (1973):987–1002.)

There are interesting correlations between motor and sensory organizations and also some differences that need to be considered. We have seen that sensory performance reaches its summit in conscious awareness of the external world of which it tries to build up an image, whereas motor perfection in the end implies suppression of the conscious component in favor of automatization of the demanded actions. The pianist and the skilled typist are not conscious of what their fingers are doing as long as they are doing it according to an automatized program. The coactivated alpha and gamma motoneurons follow the instructions, and several feedback mechanisms (eye, ear, muscle spindles, skin, tendon, and joint organs) report on perfection and elicit error correction, conscious or unconscious, as the case may be.

Learning motor acts by secret automatic routes is strikingly illustrated by some patients with severe and persistent anterograde amnesia, which implies inability to store or retrieve new memories (Scoville and Milner; Teuber).[169] When trained to do tracking tasks or to learn minor drawing tests, these patients may acquire increasingly greater skill from day to day without ever remembering that they have seen the apparatus to which they return day after day. Thus a virtually normal capacity for motor learning may coexist with absence of conscious sensory learning. Some aspects of learning and memory will be discussed in Chapter 10.

Visual learning is largely conscious learning, whereas the proprioceptive accompaniments of motor skill do not at all, or to a much lesser degree, reach conscious awareness. Proprioceptive information is not well perceived. We possess length-recording muscle receptors (the spindles) but no percept of muscle length, only a general awareness of tension. Nevertheless, proprioceptive feedback is important in movement.

Experiments on 20 sec short-term memory have shown that blind kinesthetic learning for moving a lever at a given distance leads to considerable forgetting, although conscious visual locations of position are easily remembered over that time (Posner).[170] However, conscious awareness is the more adaptable mechanism and so, if visual remembering is disturbed by an interpolated purposive act such as a verbalized task, it erases the original engram when inserted in the pause between checkings. By contrast, such interference leaves proprioceptive learning undisturbed.

In creating a body image, the child in fumbling is faced with the necessity of integrating information from many different sources: (1) visual, the most important contribution in normal people; (2) vestibular, from two ears, each with five different sense organs; (3) sensory endings for touch and pressure in the skin; (4) two kinds of spindle endings in most muscles, above all those around the neck, the arms, the legs, and the spine; (5) tendon organs recording tension; and (6) three types of endings in a large number of joints. Schematically speaking, information from at least twenty subsystems is needed, and so there will be adjustment to 2^{20} combinations! The final result will be a body image (postural model) whose existence is demonstrated when destroyed by disease. Patients of this kind are helpless when they are asked to show parts of their body. They may be so to the extent of believing that an eye or an arm is missing when asked to point to it (Schilder).[171] The postural model is also disturbed, and they may be incapable of starting a movement. Can we ever go beyond the anecdotal description of such personal tragedies for a look at the "inside" of the organized high level integrations? I shall come to some kind of answer later.

As long as vision and hearing are excluded, most readers may willingly admit that there must exist an important subconscious organization capable of dealing with movements within the body space. But neither eye nor ear can be left outside these integrations. Both sense organs have extensive subcortical projections, and even in the monkey the kind of blindness produced by ablation of the geniculostriate projections to the visual area leaves the animal capable of visual orientation and of reaching for desirable objects (Weiskrantz).[123]

Need for Stimulus-Bound Approaches

The components of an integration can hardly be analyzed unless a beginning is made with stimulus-bound approaches. And if the problem then is taken to the level of single-cell recording, at least some kind of insight can be reached. For example, a monkey can be trained to follow the movement of a small target with an equally fast eye movement. In the hindpart (flocculus) of the cerebellum Miles and Fuller have discovered neurons that specifically respond to this velocity signal.[172] These cells are independent of head movement. The input signal is the slippage of the image across the retina. The cerebellar neurons translate this signal into a command for the brainstem motoneurons of the eye muscles to pursue the target and keep it in focus. The will enters into this operation by deciding which target should be placed into the fovea of the retina. The execution of the command is left to the automaton, and so slavish pursuit proceeds until some whim of the animal urges it to use its saccadic system—another independent mechanism—to redirect the gaze elsewhere. At the level of systems analysis the same problem recurs. There is no escape from the stimulus. Specific systems or organs are engaged in selecting the speed at which any movement is supposed to be performed. These deliver the instructions to the motor apparatus (Bouisset and Lestienne).[173] We know that there are cells in the so-called basal ganglia (pallidum) which preferentially respond to slow movements (DeLong and Strick).[174] It has furthermore been found that cooling one of the cerebellar nuclei (dentatus) slows down movement (Conrad and Brooks).[174] Such cells are likely to be concerned in issuing the instructions regarding the speed of a muscular act. Such instructions are likely to be reformulated within the cortical motor area after a preliminary elaboration of instructions in the cerebellum and the basal ganglia. We are familiar with the presence of cells in the motor area whose activity precedes motor acts and demands force or velocity of application of force from the motor apparatus in the spinal cord (Evarts).[166] But independently of whether force at this or that velocity of performance is urged upon an organism by external stimuli or is ordered from the store by an act of willing, the same executive mechanisms are likely to be employed.

Purposive Sensorimotor Integrations

Motor action takes place within a sensory envelope whose presence and stability is constantly confirmed by daily renewal of the same experiences. This perpetual confirmation has created the neural organizations engineering the constancies and frameworks of reference discussed in

Chapter 6. These developments are taken into account in motor activity. Within the surrounding space such as a room we move with the greatest ease between objects whose size is constant rather than variable with the retinal image. Because our movements are scaled to this invariant world, it should be possible to detect cells in the cortex that somehow have the properties of coordinating the motor and sensory spheres. In a sense the pyramidal cells of the motor cortex and the motoneurons of the spinal cord represent stimuli and movements combined. But, in looking for cells inserted into our established organizations for movement within spatial coordinates, a more sophisticated response pattern is required than that of pyramidal cells and motoneurons which deliver force and rate of change of force to commands from elsewhere.

The signs of the postulated sophistication are somehow related to varieties of behavior, and by accepting behavioral criteria we have chosen to adopt a number of psychological concepts such as motivation, attention, interest, or demand. Alternatively, we have abandoned the urge to use whatever means are at our disposal for making experimental observations meaningful. Units within the parietal cortex exemplify the required properties. This part of the brain lies behind the sensory area and above the temporal lobe. Clinical experience testifies to the complex and variegated symptomatology of parietal destructive processes (Critchley).[175] Though the threshold for skin sensations may be little altered, there are striking defects in the synthesis, interpretation, differentiation, and comparison of the elementary sensory experiences. "Touch and vision are partners when it comes to affording us information as to the nature, physical properties and identity of objects around us" (Critchley, p. 109). They also contribute to the building-up of the body image and the coordinates of the postural model. Postural loss and defects in recognition of passive joint movements are seen with parietal lesions. The body image is needed for movement. Single-cell analysis again has shown a way of closing in on these problems (Mountcastle and his colleagues; Hyvärinen and Poranen).[176]

One of the cell types in the parietal area could not be activated by any passively delivered stimulus but was fired in movements aimed at securing something the monkey desired like food. For this purpose it had to close a switch or pull a lever. Outwardly similar, active movements of an aggressive or aversive character did not excite these neurons. The cue used for detection of the desired object was unimportant—it might be visual, tactile, or acoustic; nor was the trajectory by which the goal was reached or the length of the time of expectation after the first warning signal of any significance. Thus the real stimulus appeared to be anticipation of what the reward was good for. The cellular discharge actually ended before the movement itself was completed. Because the neuron began firing in anticipation, the movement could not have been the cause of the discharge; it seems more likely that it was a consequence of the internal stimulus taking a routine course and using the required movement from the available repertoire. The significant point appears to be that the neuron was imbedded in an internal organization for signaling something like "Eureka, this is worth going for," a kind of purpose detector related by the affective quality of the stimulus to the movement signaling accomplishment.

In another part of the parietal lobe, Mountcastle's group discovered neurons that fired when the monkey became interested in a visually fixated object within reach. The fir-

ing of these cells diminished when the object was moved
farther away from the animal. The three discernible components integrated into the discharge were (1) successful
fixation, that is, the object had to be foveally located; (2) it
had to be within arm's length; and (3) it had to be interesting. These neurons also discharged when the animal was
grooming itself. If the visual cue was blocked, the cell was
silenced. Similarly it failed to respond if the target fell within a part of the visual field that was prevented from picking
up the object by fixation. Like the neurons previously described, this type also required motivation for a definite
purpose, but it differed from the former by being tightly
bound to the act of fixation of a visual target at a short distance. Its explorative character was directed and restricted
to the immediately surrounding space.

A third type of neuron in the parietal lobe was a sensitive
indicator of steady joint position. Many of the neurons related to joint position were more active during active movements than when the limbs were passively displaced.

Other types of neurons have been found in this region
but cannot be discussed here. As an assembly of different
properties they help us to understand why an authority in
the clinical field has been compelled to state: "To seek to
establish a formula of normal parietal function is largely a
vain and meaningless pursuit, however attractive" (Critchley, p. 410).[175] Partly, of course, a pathological process may
not be restricted to the parietal lobes, but it seems more important that localized integrative acts end up in single neurons combining information and action in many different
ways. A cortical lobe, or even a cortical field of considerable
homogeneity from the histological point of view, contains
highly differentiated cell patterns. These are not easily
distinguished by conceptual subdivisions based on the re-

sources of our language. Disease may hit them indiscrimi-
nately. Nevertheless the clinician somehow adumbrates
gross function, as does Critchley: "The peculiar role of the
parietal lobe—or lobes—in the building-up of the postural
schema of the body leads to an important association with
corporeal awareness, imagery and memory. Hence the appearance of unusual disorders of the body-image with
parietal disease" (p. 411).

Active vs. Passive Sensorimotor Activity

It has been briefly mentioned that the central nervous system is organized for active selection of the stimuli whose
effects it for some reason or other wants to incorporate—
that is, use for its integrations—while rejecting the rest.
When conscious, we can of course decide what the selection
should be, but most of the acts of selecting are carried out
by teleologically organized processes over which we do not
retain control. We encountered such processes when discussing adaptability in Chapter 3.

The experience of behavioral physiologists from animal
work is that selecting and interpreting information to establish visually guided motor activity requires that the actual movements of the limbs are both made and seen to be
made. Without self-produced movements the necessary coordinations do not develop in kittens (Held and Hein).[177]
And a large number of physiological experiments show
that improvement of performance takes place when active
movements are substituted for passive ones. In the previous section I mentioned the single cells in the parietal
cortex that only responded to active movements at the
joints. An interesting case from this point of view was reported by Lashley in 1917.[178] He investigated the motor

behavior of a man with a gunshot injury that had left one leg without sensitivity to movement at the knee joint. The blindfolded patient was unable to detect large passive swings of the nonsentient leg, but when told to swing it himself, he judged about the extent of movement with remarkable accuracy. The finding can be explained in several ways, but it is used here merely to illustrate the significance of active versus passive sensorimotor activity.

Vision, with its 2 million afferent fibers in the optic nerves and its large cortical representation, tends to dominate over proprioceptive and skin senses. If the arm is swung up and down at the elbow joint in the dark, and, suddenly, a flash illuminates the limb, the subject feels his limb to be at rest in the position at which it was caught by the flash (Hagbarth).[179]

Principles Applied in Explanations

The preceding references to some properly analyzed sensorimotor integrations in single neurons and to the role of self-activation for the development of motor skills in orientation have been chosen to illustrate essential steps toward understanding sensorimotor integrations. At one time it was commonly held that the fundamental principle behind cortical operations was merely one of association, and from this period stems the name of "association areas" for the fields that did not represent direct projections from sense organs or else were motor in character. Association may also be used in the vague general sense of standing for the fact that motor and sensory events *are* associated in the phenomena described. But the old association theory, in addition, implied an explanation by association caused by proximity in time and space of objective stimuli or events, which by virtue of this coexistence became semipermanently coupled in memory. This notion balanced emphasis wrongly.

The trend of my discourse points in a different direction. Little importance has been attached to the basic coexistence in time and space for the formation of associations. Instead I have emphasized that (1) from simultaneously available information the purposive brain selects what it finds biologically useful; (2) in this way it employs its billions of neurons to create unique cellular organs of high specificity combining information from various sources with action; (3) such organs are mobilized by injecting into them components that we describe in such psychological terms as motivation, interest, anger, demand, or accomplishment—in short, relevance for some biological purpose. From the evolutionary standpoint "teleonomic purposiveness" is involved in addition to the true teleological purposiveness discussed in Chapter 3. These factors are more important than sheer simultaneity in time or space. Most simultaneous events—luckily—go unnoticed.

By far the most revealing information on the tasks of interpretation and action in our purposive brain has come from the study of single neurons, many examples of which have been given in this and previous chapters. Nevertheless it is evident that the individual neuron only represents an elaborate cellular organization within the cortex. Such structures could be columnar organizations (mentioned in Chapter 6) whose existence repeatedly has been confirmed for the visual and tactile spheres.[108] Mountcastle and his colleagues saw something of these also in the parietal cortex, but they were also compelled to introduce the notion of block formation to account for the orderly presence of specific types of neurons.

At the level of the visual primary projections it is possible to speak of detector or trigger features, but this does not help us much to understand the sophisticated neurons that connect vision to doing. Consider integrated conditions for such activity as "reachability" of an object together with its capability of evoking the anticipation of pleasure leading to the combination of movement with interest; for these neurons the object also had to be fixated within the fovea. This means that whatever detector mechanisms were available for an optimal definition of the object are also likely to have been actively employed. But having delivered their special contribution to the integrated act—to help distinguish and identify the target with maximal perfection—their role was over. Once and for all the object *was* detected. This elementary function was incorporated in the integration as one of the prerequisites for action. The rest of the neuronal properties of the cellular organization to which these neurons belong are held together by realizing some purposive demand and by notifying its accomplishment.

Central sites for recording pleasure are known (Olds and Milner)[180] as well as centers for arousal. For this reason it seems likely that the response of the parietal neurons would require intact connections with these sites. Even if we cannot trace the precise pathways involved in the creation of complex, highly individualized responses of cellular units located beyond the specific sensory projection areas, we can rely on anatomy to supply whatever combinations physiological and behavioral facts might require. No analysis is ever likely to end up with anatomy as the great stumbling block in the way of progress. More often than not we shall find it difficult to understand the purpose that provides biological relevance to a response found in these hierarchic tiers.

Attention, Demand, and Behavior

In considering motor activity in the highly encephalized primates including ourselves, terms and concepts that belong to the topmost hierarchic stratum are usually introduced into the text.[181] Up to a point we can neglect such aspects of movement control and consider the recording of properties of muscles and nerve cells in joint action and the elucidation of wiring diagrams, disregarding the question of why the recorded events take place in the particular manner observed. Such work will often furnish the neurophysiologist with significant knowledge. But then for over a hundred years experimental physiology has been interested in voluntary movement and today, when by an act of willing a subject demands force and a prescribed velocity of performance, it is possible to translate demand into firing rates of motoneurons and muscles and to some extent even into discharge rates of groups of single neurons in the cortex.[182] From these data as a starting point one can proceed "vertically" upward or downward in the hierarchic cascade of strata.

However, by such experiments one has neither explained will as such nor its immense range of demand, its relation to attention, nor its dependence on motivation. Some idea of will power can be obtained by pitting a demanded set of instructions against automatic segmental mechanisms and determining to what extent the latter can be overridden. Both for theoretical and for clinical purposes such studies of the act of willing or demanding are of considerable importance. Nevertheless will and demand remain what they always were— psychological concepts required in the study of behavior. More will be said about such questions at the end of the next chapter.

10
Aims and Limits of Explaining and Understanding

The scientific terms of "explanation" are "not necessarily immediately in evidence. They have to be discovered, and their discovery involves our taking the phenomena to be explained at the right level of analysis and with the right conceptual framework . . . the correlations on one level are explained by those on a deeper level in a way which shows their relation to other possible outcomes." (Charles Taylor, *The Explanation of Purposive Behaviour*, Cambridge University Press, 1970, pp. 52–53.)[183]

Integration, Models, and Hypotheses

"Integration" has been mentioned repeatedly and been defined as interaction for a purpose. Some comments are needed to indicate the limitations of this concept as a scientific tool. It shares with other concepts the general property of being most useful when something can be formulated as a hypothesis actually featuring the integration. An example is reciprocal innervation as part of the mechanism of stepping. A model of this act represents a further concretization of the scientific hypothesis and so, whether good or faulty, it is a step on the road to understanding what one has observed and thought. But even if our model is the best we can design, it does not necessarily summarize everything known about a given set of data. The designer may have to be content with a scheme embodying some highly significant features of the findings. When these are modeled, the major aim tends to be the experimenter's desire to test interpretations by a concretization that can be used for prediction and at its best for a quantitative control of the factors involved.

When Sherrington in 1904 delivered his Silliman Lectures and published them in 1906 (*Integrative Action of the Nervous System*), the term "integration" entered the vocabulary of scientific neurology.[96] At the time his emphasis was on action exemplified by reflexes. He pointed out that reflexes had to be purposive and "the purpose of a reflex seems as legitimate and urgent an object for natural inquiry as the purpose of colouring of an insect or blossom." The actual experimental work concentrated on the properties of the "final common path," which was represented by the single motoneuron whose membrane integrated the inputs. The analysis concentrated on the mechanisms whereby excitatory and inhibitory processes, initiated by different inputs, interacted to grade the output of a pool of motoneurons for different purposes. From this starting point we have seen work expand downward and upward: downward to the study of the properties of synapses and cell membranes in chemical and physical terms, and upward to the highly complex circuits (wiring diagrams) engaged—as we have reason to believe—in selecting the teleologically appropriate motoneuronal responses.

A useful wiring diagram is essentially a little computer and so has a purpose at its own level. Circuit analysis concurrently represents the best we can do in modeling an integration. However, in hierarchic systems there is likewise a corresponding hierarchy of purposes, which is well put by Polanyi when he says: "the integration of items of a lower level so as to predict their possible meaning in a higher context may be beyond the range of our integrative powers" (p. 1312).[72]

An example is indicated to follow up these reflections. Figure 10.1 illustrates one of the best analyzed wiring diagrams we possess: the segmental mechanism of reciprocal innervation. The primary muscle spindle afferents, whose impulses α γ Ia arrive from the knee extensor (quadriceps), reach the motoneurons of their own muscle monosynaptically and send a branch to an interneuron I, which is inhibitory on the antagonist flexor muscle PBSt. Thus, when the agonist extensor is excited, the antagonist flexor is reciprocally inhibited by the same α γ Ia afferent input. There is a corresponding organization for the flexor as agonist on the extensor as antagonist so that we see only half of the complete diagram in the figure. One clearly purposive element of this circuit is to serve alternating flexor and extensor contractions in stepping. The quadriceps motoneuron has a recurrent collateral that excites the Renshaw cell, an interneuron with inhibitory effect upon the muscle's motoneurons. This R cell is also inhibitory on the interneuron I that mediates the reciprocal inhibition. This means that the greater the output firing rate of the quadriceps motoneuron M, the greater also the excitatory state of R and consequently its two inhibitory effects—one on quadriceps itself and the other on the interneuron I that mediates antagonist inhibition. Thus both agonist excitation and antagonist inhibition are provided with a common output-operated feedback loop curbing hyperactivity and preventing both motoneurons from reaching extreme degrees of excitation or inhibition, all done by the elegant expedient of recurrent inhibition (Lundberg).[155]

Simple and satisfying as this specimen of a well-analyzed integration seems, it can also be used to illustrate the limitations of thinking in terms of wiring diagrams. The two interneurons R and I are both in turn controlled by a large number of spinal afferents and, most significantly, by several supraspinal pathways such as those of the cortical motor area. Either or both interneurons can thus be excited or inhibited. Assume that such a supraspinal pathway excites the R cell. The effect would be to oppose reciprocal innervation and balance the segmental mechanisms in favor of cocontractions of agonist and antagonist. The same effect could be obtained by a supraspinal excitation of both motoneurons or by inhibition of the I cell preventing the inhibition of the antagonist. Again, in stepping it would be advantageous for the alternating flexor-extensor movements if the R cell were inhibited so that the full reciprocal effect from the I cell were free to operate. This is actually known to be the case (Feldman and Orlovsky).[184]

Obviously, with the large number of controls not insert-

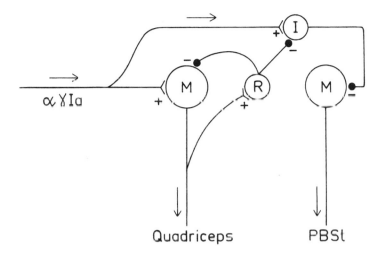

Quadriceps   PBSt

10.1. Diagram to show reciprocal innervation. The alpha gamma Ia input from the muscle spindles excites the quadriceps muscle's motoneuron (M) and inhibits that of the mm. posterior biceps-semitendinosus across interneuron I. The interneuron R, excited on the output line of quadriceps, inhibits its own motoneuron as well as the interneuron I, thus curbing excitation of quadriceps and inhibition of PBSt. From Ragnar Granit, *Brain*, 98, Part IV, pp. 531–556.

ed here of both R and I, exceedingly fine adjustments of agonist and antagonist contributions to a motor act are possible. All are integrations (that is, interactions for a purpose), but at this point we come up against the characteristic limitations of vertebrate wiring diagrams. The number of permutations for every possible purpose is without bound.

Under the circumstances, what have we explained and understood? At the back of it all is our basic understanding of the role of interneurons, namely, that they exist to realize the high degree of adaptability with respect to environmental variables discussed in Chapter 3. Furthermore, we have understood what kind of a mechanism is available at the segmental level for this end. It can never become our final goal to account for every conceivable possibility. The wiring diagrams should be regarded as constraints or boundary conditions that have to be fitted into broad generalizations such as the existence of reciprocal innervation, alpha-gamma linkage with its implications discussed in Chapter 7, or stabilization by feedback. In this context they represent real understanding of neural operations. Circuit analysis is necessary also for cybernetic approaches to control problems (see next section). Integrative thinking and cybernetics have a common interest in wiring diagrams as part of the hardware.

When the term integration is used in the way exemplified by the purposive cells mentioned in the previous chapter, it may sometimes be possible to predict the existence and general features of the operative circuit. This was the case with the cerebellar cells activated in proportion to velocity of eye movements, though actually featuring the circuit here would require more anatomical detail than it is possible to introduce. In the case of the parietal cells a number of important ingredients of their integrated activity were defined, but of the two questions, "how come" and "what for," only the latter received a reasonably convincing answer.

Cybernetic Explanations

Inasmuch as cybernetics is the science of regulation and control, it has had a long clandestine existence in physiology, because the latter science has always been concerned with regulated and controlled processes.[185,186] Ewald Hering in 1868 wrote an article on the "Self-steering of respiration through nervus vagus," a mechanism presupposing regulation by feedback. Cannon's term "homeostasis" (1924)[186] covered a concept developed by Claude Bernard around 1878 which implied that a constant internal milieu within an organism is preserved by a number of compensatory feedback activities. Sherrington's discussion of the stretch reflex as an antigravity response, counteracting lengthening of a leg extensor by a reflex shortening of it, was based on the leading cybernetic idea of negative feedback.

The conceptual generalizations of cybernetics with their mathematical treatment of circuits including the full information theory (Wiener;[34] Shannon;[70] Harmon[165]) arrived as late as the 1940s.[187] These contributions held out an enticing promise of opening up a new world of final explanations of the properties of the nervous system and its great computer: our thinking and feeling brain.

The disappointment we register today derives from the understanding that cybernetics is but one approach among many others, highly useful when a reasonably simple wiring diagram can be found, but by no means any final "open sesame." This is not because neural circuits fail to obey the boundary conditions laid down in the rules of regulation science, but rather because such circuits as we have seen only rarely can be lifted out of their context for isolated treatment guided by cybernetic rules. The nervous system is organized as a comparator and synthesizer with hierarchic stratification of excitatory or inhibitory controls. The consequences of an enormous redundancy—not reproduced by any computer—are incalculable. For such reasons mathematical circuit analysis is limited to model-making with simplified wiring diagrams, useful insofar as the approximations approach some fraction of reality. An example of a successful application is provided by the relatively simple pupillary reflex to light (Stark).[188]

In Chapter 7 I mentioned the difficulties alluded to by the stretch reflex. Ostensibly this reflex offered a simple enough wiring diagram and so it was thought to be fully comprehensible in terms of cybernetics. However, the science of physiology, patiently advancing in its own tortuous, experimental fashion, gradually brought forth numerous complications, most of which could be regarded as essential for understanding the role of the stretch reflex in movement and posture. Thus the stretch reflex was found to be regulated by the size of motoneurons, the duration of their after-hyperpolarizations, recurrent inhibition, and tendon-reflex inhibition. It was found to need the support of differentially biased interneurons as well as that of static and dynamic gamma motor fibers regulating the sensitivity of the stretch receptors (muscle spindles). These motor fibers in turn were shown to be ruled by numerous supraspinal stations according to the needs of the moment. And ultimately in some cases the stretch reflex acting in load compensation has been demonstrated to require a loop operating through the motor cortex. In this formidable expansion of our understanding of this one reflex alone, the least important contribution came from the application of mathematical circuit analysis. More examples are unnecessary. Once more it turns out that hierarchic organizations of the degree of complexity of our nervous system require understanding at each level of what the hierarchies themselves are meant to supply. Communication mathematics is of little help in this regard. Consider, for instance, the properties of the parietal cells, mentioned in Chapter 9. These synthetic neurons, which combine a number of features required for action, are truly purposive cells, and the communication engineer's concept of information measured in "bits per second" does not add one bit to the understanding of their design and specific sensitivities.

Does this amount to a repudiation of cybernetics? Emphatically no. I merely want to indicate its limitations. It should be gratefully admitted that cybernetics has clarified thinking in regulation terms and has provided biology with a number of highly instructive operational terms such as "gain," "stability," "gating," "feedback," "feed-forward," and "redundancy," some of which have been introduced into previous chapters. Even when used without their full quantitative implications, they have influenced our attitude toward the experimental material. Just as in mathematics the concepts of integration and differentiation have made scientists recognize physical and physiological events as being of either type, so the concepts of regulation science have drawn attention to fundamental modes of nervous action classifiable in cybernetic categories. And why should not this be so? Somehow our thinking must reflect the properties of our central nervous system.

It might be added that experts in communication theory and cybernetics, like Machin and Harmon, are more cautious in their judgments about the value of communication science than enthusiastic amateurs from the biological camp. Machin stated: "By the time the physiologist has reached the stage of fitting the elements of the transfer function to the structure of his biological system, he is beyond the point where feedback theory can help him. A knowledge of current engineering techniques may guide analogistic thinking, and some idea of what is not possible may prevent wrong guesses" (p. 444).[187]

Localization and Function

Previous chapters have raised the problem of localization and function from different aspects, ultimately carrying it to the level of single neurons for which it can be stated most succinctly. The exquisite specificity with which some of these cells synthesize information from different sources and initiate complex motor activities makes one wonder whether our experimental inventiveness suffices for discovering everything that a cell in the interpreting cortex can respond to and do. Our repertoire of tests may well be too stereotyped for the cellular homunculus.

The most general conclusion that can be drawn is that such highly talented neurons receive information from many other brain regions and have access to command neurons for specific motor acts using segmentally organized responses within the spinal cord. If one such highly specific neuron were killed, would we lose the function that it has mastered to such perfection? Almost certainly not.

The basic redundancy of the neural organizations is not likely to have left significant operations dependent on a single cell. Blocks of them do the same or much the same thing. Lashley, working with rats in 1930, noted that large portions of the cortex could be removed without significantly altering their behavior in a maze.[189] Similar results have since been obtained by others (Doty; Weiskrantz).[123] In studies of visually guided acts of discrimination in the cat, sectioning of most of the optic tract produced only small impairment of performance, but in this case the accessory visual tract, normally perhaps rather unimportant, may have been responsible for a substitution.[190] The animals also adopt different strategies (eye and head movements) to compensate for the loss.

Man, at a higher stage of cortical development, is likely to possess still more highly specified neurons, greater redundancy, and more intricate circuits joining many more cortical sites than animals at a lower level. It does not seem probable that neurophysiology will ever succeed in tracing all the relevant connections leading up to a purposive movement. The limit of our understanding seems to be reached with the specification of integrations within a single cell. An alternative way of advancing such problems is to turn to systems analysis. At all stages of interpretation our present ignorance of the chemistry and circuitry of engram formation remains a formidable obstacle in the way of progress.

It is true that at the moment localization of any definable function may seem to be dominated by the topological point of view. Yet in the end a purely cartographic map of functions cannot be our final aim. One must hope and believe that components of insight into new and unexpected roles of localization will be revealed by continued patient experimentation. This at least is the way that neurophysiology often has reached many of its most important results. At a certain point the perspective has suddenly widened to permit understanding such previously unrelatable observations that were intelligently restricted to the momentarily soluble. The same general attitude is adopted by the physicists trying to penetrate the mysteries of an ever-increasing number of particles within the atom.

One of the oldest findings in localization physiology is the discovery of the language areas of the brain (Broca and Wernicke).[191] The old clinical work made it probable that language as spoken, written, heard, and understood was localized to the left hemisphere. The split-brain patients, mentioned in Chapter 5, provided a crucial test of this hypothesis. It is now known that communication by language in most people is virtually restricted to the left hemisphere, though something is understood by its right partner. Transferred to animals, the split-brain technique has become an important tool in the search for other hemispherical asymmetries.

A function to be localized is dependent on our use of language to supply a name for it from experience. The selected name need not necessarily cover anything morphologically or physiologically homogeneous, or we may not see the reason why certain functions are interconnected. Rather safe choices of functions refer to such states as attention (arousal)[192], sleep, hunger, and thirst. All these functions are to some extent corticalized, but they are decisively controlled by the phylogenetically old parts of the brain common to all vertebrates. Governing circuits of the sleep-wakefulness cycle, for instance, are found in "old" parts of the brain (anterior hypothalamus, basal forebrain, and the posterior hypothalamus) but in this issue the great-

er problem of the levels of activation required for different
kinds of behavior looms large, according to Moruzzi.[85] The
stereotactic technique of introducing stimulating needles
into the brain for localization purposes (Horsley-Clarke
technique, used by Hess, Ranson, and numerous followers)
has revealed a wealth of localized subcortical functions
such as thirst, hunger, pleasure, anger, sleep, and specific
movements.

Well-defined states are often represented by systems
such as those controlling sleep and wakefulness occupying
sites in different regions. Knowledge of such systems is of
considerable clinical importance. They are often chemically homogeneous with regard to synaptic transmitter substances (see the next section), and if they cannot be so
defined, physiological analysis becomes difficult. Faulty
conceptualization may be involved. It is for example an
open question how far we can go in the following case (Pribram and McGuinness).[193] Three systems are assumed:
control of *arousal*; controls of *activation*, defined as tonic
readiness to respond; and controls coordinating arousal
with activation and requiring *effort* that leads to maintenance of attention. Do these categories represent a useful or
merely a heroic attempt at conceptualization in search of
morphological equivalents? Time will tell. Arousal itself
has been well defined and much studied (Jasper, Magoun,
Moruzzi). Its origin is in an extensive system of basally
located neurons.

Surgical removal of a region whose function we want to
know may not provide a final answer, because often it will
merely tell us what the brain can do despite the loss instead
of telling us what the lost portion did. Nevertheless such
experiences have proved very useful in the identification
of functions, and now they also serve as an antidote against

prematurely assigning too great a role to the best analyzed single neurons of the cortex.

Engram Formation

No subject in present-day brain science has attracted more students than learning, that is, engram formation and hence memory. The experimenters come from psychology, behavioral sciences, neurophysiology, clinical medicine, and biochemistry. In this vast domain volumes would be needed merely to review the pertinent literature.[194]

Clearly everything that has been said in previous chapters about the properties of individual neurons, as elucidated by testing, has presupposed modeling by memory traces, those most elusive engrams. Perceptions are continuously matched against stored experience and motor acts make use of stored programs. And yet remembering cannot be explained in any but the most general terms. It all reduces to two statements: (1) engrams must be based on circuitry transmitting information in an organized manner, and (2) to most workers memory seems inexplicable unless produced by chemical changes mediated by the synaptic apparatus.

So far the biochemical evidence has been general rather than specific, but the most significant feature of a stored engram, next to its durability, is its individual character. The important contributions have come from the fields of psychology and behavior joining forces. As to physiology, I tend to agree with Broadbent who maintains that "there seems to be no sign as yet of a link between physiology and psychology of this field" (p. 349).[194] Clinical medicine, to be sure, provides an interesting contact, but it is chiefly concerned with localization rather than with the physiological nature of the mechanism.

For over a century psychologists have amassed data on memory, and their findings have been a permanent source of inspiration for modern behavioral studies. Clinical neurology has helped to elaborate two of the major concepts—short-term memory and long-term memory. There is general agreement on the existence of a "simple iconic store, from which later and more complex processes select certain items for encoding" (Broadbent).[194] However, even short-term memory seems to involve quite complex processes, as recently shown with the split-brain subjects (Zeidel and Sperry);[195] these patients differed from normal people and epileptics in having marked impairment of short-term memory despite otherwise good performance in tests for intelligence level. Thus some interhemispheric interaction seems to be required for normal short-term memory. Many clinical cases can be adduced in support of preserved intelligence despite loss of recent memory.

To illustrate preserved short-term memory despite lack of capacity for transferring items into the long-term store, I shall take a famous patient who for two decades has been studied with great analytical skill and much perseverance, particularly by Brenda Milner.[196] Several reports, preceded by her own, have recently been collected in an issue of *Neuropsychologia* (1968, vol. 6). This patient was successfully operated on for epilepsy by Scoville in 1953 before it was known that removal of the two temporal lobes with encroachment upon the bilateral structure on its inside, known as the hippocampus, leads to permanent loss of the capacity to make long-term engrams. What this subject has read in a magazine or a newspaper is totally forgotten after

15 minutes. The patient is still unable to find his way home from a nearby store but is quite capable of solving difficult crossword puzzles and of acquiring motor skills. He lives from moment to moment, as short-term memory is essentially unimpaired, but has also old memories with orderly retrieval.

Computers can be designed to store information and retrieve it. For these and other reasons extensive analogies based on computer science have been proposed. As to these efforts I am inclined to side with Weiskrantz when he states that these "analogies are not wrong in the sense of making false predictions about behaviour: they are simply irrelevant, the real brain has a different organization; the logical structure is different" (p. 336); therefore what is being produced is a number of "elegant irrelevancies."[197]

Systems in Balance and Release

The discussion of systems would be simplified if their homogeneity in a histochemical sense represented one single function, corresponding to a chosen term. This is rarely the case. My statement should be qualified by an example. The substances known as catecholamines have long played an important role in physiology. To this group belong, for instance, epinephrine (adrenaline) and norepinephrine (noradrenaline). Large-scale histochemical identification of catecholamines began with the discovery (Eränkö; Falck and Hillarp)[140] of a fluorescence technique of staining them in situ and sectioning the tissues for microscopical analysis. One system traced by this technique contained dopamine; its distribution is illustrated in Figure 10.2 from the rat's brain (Ungerstedt).[198] It occupies much space in the subcortical brain (substantia nigra to neostriatum).

DOPAMINE

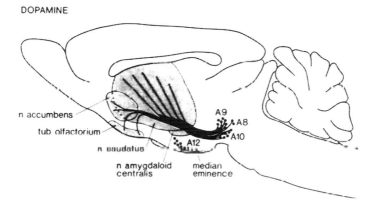

10.2. Sagittal projection of the dopaminergic pathway in the rat's brain. The stripes indicate nerve terminal areas. From Urban Ungerstedt, *Acta Physiologica Scandinavica* (1971), Suppl. 367.

The dopamine in this system can be removed by intra-cerebral injection of a highly specific antagonist or by electrocoagulation of its axons. A complex pathological picture develops. The animal shows loss of exploratory behavior, inability to initiate action, subnormal motor activity, and inability to feed and drink. This dopaminergic system therefore governs a number of functions in a critical manner. The results are of great interest in clinical medicine because lack of cellular dopamine in the same sites characterizes Parkinson's disease in which similar defects of motor control occur.[199] The patients are rigid, shaky, and voluntary action is delayed and slowed down. A number of those patients can now be cured by supplying the missing dopamine as L-dopa tablets. (For a review, see Hornykiewicz.)[199]

It is a curious fact that despite the existence of several motor systems the loss of this particular one should disturb motor activity in such a profound fashion. Removal of the total motor cortex of the rat would be less serious than Ungerstedt's experiments; we have seen in Chapter 3 that the nervous system is highly adaptable and can adjust itself to loss of tissue. As already mentioned, it is possible to remove an entire large organ such as the cerebellum without noticing equally radical changes of motor behavior. In fact, irregularities are detectable only by subtle tests provided an animal is in possession of full visual control compensating for the loss.

The cerebellum consists of small and large cells, the latter (Purkinje cells) responsible for the output to the cerebellar (inside) nuclei. The connections and synaptic effects of the small cells are known but their basic role unknown. The small cells can be selectively destroyed by X-raying the cerebellum at an early developmental stage, which leaves a cerebellum of large cells alone (Altman and Anderson).[200] These animals never learn to move normally.

These examples show that disturbing a nicely set balance point within a system may be more dangerous than complete removal of it. The general concept by which such facts are explained is known as "release." Historically it goes back at least to Setchenow (1863).[201] Release does not tell us very much more than that the balance between interconnected systems is important and that upsetting it may lead to an undesirable preponderance of one particular component over the rest. In particular, inhibitions are required to counteract excitations that when released from this constraint may run amok. In a cascading development of elaborated acts or percepts, there may be sites in the pathway that, within a volume of the order of a square millimeter, are carrying extremely relevant messages, neatly balanced for a purpose, be it sensory or motor. A small destruction may then lead to dramatic effects while large cortical ablations proceed unnoticed.

For example, surgery is another cure of Parkinson's disease, now largely superseded by the L-dopa treatment. The rigid, fully conscious patient is seated in a chair with his head clamped while a needle, insulated except at the tip, is directed to a critical site in the thalamus. The brain itself is not sensitive to pain. During coagulation of a small spot in one of the thalamic nuclei, the patient feels his rigidity slowly melt away and he rises relieved from the chair, feeling that he has had a dramatic experience of deliverance.

The thalamus is a structure in the uppermost region below the cortex. It contains some of the most essential cellular nuclei for preliminary integration of what the cortex needs for its various motor as well as sensory activities. The sensory input runs through its synaptic organization, and all the cortical fields have loops to and from it. There are connections also with the cerebellum and the basal ganglia. We know far too little about the role of the thalamus. The reason may well be neglect of purposive thinking. Most neurophysiologists are happier with a clean "reductionist" physicochemical approach and look with disdain on experimental work designed for the elucidation of purpose. Clearly it is safer to remain with problems that can be solved by conventional means rather than go for the purpose of something observed in the manner of von Frisch dealing with the dance of the honeybee (Chapter 1).

Lessons from Studying Simple Organisms

In a sense, primitive organisms present the experimenter with models applicable to complex creatures. They have chiefly been of service in our attempts to understand physical and chemical events at synapses and membranes. The reason for this is Nature's tendency to go on improving early inventions rather than try totally new solutions. One of the best examples is the nerve impulse. In the squid there is a giant nerve fiber nearly 1 mm in diameter (J. Z. Young), as against the 0.020 mm of the largest vertebrate nerve fibers. It is possible to insert a microelectrode into this giant fiber to measure both potential and resistance across the nerve membrane (Cole; Hodgkin and A. F. Huxley).[202] A technique was developed for studying the action potential (the nerve impulse) in terms of ionic transport and permeability changes that made it possible to account for the impulse quantitatively by the ionic theory of Hodgkin and Huxley. When later electronic developments created means for testing this theory without entering the inside of a nerve fiber (Dodge and Frankenhaeuser),[203] the same theory and the same equation with only slight modifications was also proved to be valid for the single vertebrate nerve fiber. Interesting aspects of synaptic action in the snail (*Aplysia*) have also had repercussions in the field of vertebrate physiology (within which the original ideas were conceived). This is perhaps not so surprising; nerve cells, membranes, synapses, and transmitter substances are very ancient biological inventions of Nature's. These basic mechanisms do not differ fundamentally from species to species in the phylum.

Less commonly useful are the wiring diagrams established by invertebrate research. I have mentioned an important exception, Hartline's study of lateral inhibition between the retinal cells in the eye of the horseshoe crab *Limulus*.[38] This type of negative feedback serving contrast and stabilization of the outgoing discharge recurs in many places in the vertebrate central nervous system. In the latter its best-known version is the inhibition through the R cell of the recurrent collateral of the motoneuron. Also in *Limulus* the inhibition is recurrent in the sense that it lies on the output side of the retinal cells on which it acts. In *Limulus*, however, the inhibition is direct, whereas in the spinal cord one immediately encounters the characteristic complication of a higher type of nervous system. In traversing the R cell (Figure 10.1) the degree of inhibition is largely modified by numerous pathways biasing the cell.

At the level of the spiders there is a sense organ in the moving limb that, like the muscle spindle of the vertebrates, is controlled from above (Cohen),[204] but this organization was discovered after the basic principle already had been established in the mammalian preparation (Chapter 7). And this, in fact, is the more common experience: the leading role has been played by classical mammalian physiology elaborating concepts and mechanisms that later have been applied in invertebrate studies. Thus, for instance, the entire physiology of synaptic action (Sherrington;[96] Bernard Katz;[137] Eccles[28]) was developed with the aid of vertebrate preparations. The younger science of invertebrate physiology followed this lead, in the end making significant contributions of its own (Arvanitaki; Tauc; Kandel).[205] A solution of the chemical aspects of memory may well ultimately be achieved within invertebrate physiology.

The hierarchic organization of the nervous system prevents invertebrate studies from ever contributing much to the understanding of the mode of action of the mammalian brain and spinal cord beyond the level of the previous examples. Too much should not be made to rest on analogies. They can be very misleading. We shall always be compelled to live with the complexities of primate neurophysiology and the consciousness of man. For instance, when evolutionary pressure has produced eyes in both squids and squirrels necessitating focusing devices and retinas, the functions are analogous, not homologous, at least not beyond the level of the pigment photochemistry that determines the spectral sensitivity to light.

The Psychophysiological Approach

It is, of course, possible to use all the concepts referring to conscious awareness, such as perception, will, interest, demand, novelty, or similarity, as "operant definitions" without mentioning the role of consciousness itself. But this would be acting in the ostrich fashion of the early behaviorists who in their "obsessive psychophobia" denied that their research had anything to do with "mind" but was—so they maintained—purely objective. "After all, consciousness in the sense of 'being aware of' is esentially a form of knowledge. Without it, observation, which every scientist including the behaviourist automatically postulates, would be impossible" (Buit, p. 237).[73]

No sooner is one—with Sherrington[62]—prepared to look on consciousness as an emergent novelty, the greatest of Nature's innumerable inventions, than it becomes imperative to regard it as a cause on a par with other causative agents, moving muscles in speech and laughter, in posture and precision grip, and thus also moving the world. In the simplest conceivable movement it is possible to grade force and speed of action by an act of will formulated as a demand by a conscious subject. There is no reason to imagine that the outside physical world as we know it through our consciously interpreted senses is the sole manifestation of energetic relationships. The will and skill that have landed a man on the moon cannot be regarded as negligible objects of independent study, convinced though one be that the hierarchic superstratum of conscious awareness does not differ from any intermediate hierarchic tier in being somehow traceable as physiological hardware down to the very bottom of reductionism.

Furthermore, accepting the validity of hierarchic reasoning presupposes that at each level new teleological explanations will be required. A lower stratum in the hierarchy can never fully explain the raison d'être of the higher stratum above it. It follows that the properties of conscious awareness cannot be explained by any of the numerous physiological processes within reach of our technical prowess, even though without them consciousness is bound to fade away. This does not mean that the subhierarchic physiological processes are of no account, any more than the nerve impulse can be held to be of no account in the study of sensation. Correlations between events are always important as components of the structural knowledge science is engaged in creating. Hierarchic reasoning does, however, imply that in studying conscious events the propositions to be analyzed should be formulated in full recognition of consciousness as an independent principle manifesting itself in a causal context and representing the maximum adaptability of which an organism is capable. It is a futile occupation to hunt for structural parallelism or likenesses between the physiological processes and conscious awareness when all we can do is to establish correlations.

My first example of such correlations (in Chapter 6) dealt with the trichromatic theory of color perception and the existence of three kinds of retinal receptors representing the spectral distributions of sensitivity that were required by the theory. My last one, to end this collection of essays, concerns habituation and dishabituation.[206] Two classic examples are the mother sleeping through any kind of outside noise below the level of irritation but waking up to the lightest whimper of her child or the chief engineer of a steamer similarly habituated to the regular humming of his engine but aroused by the smallest irregularity in this rhythm.

It has not proved difficult to show by electroencephalography and other methods of electrical recording that objectively measured responses diminish by repetition of a stimulus and are revived by a slight change in the stimulus parameters. Thus habituation and dishabituation are embedded in the general neural fabric of reactivity, rather than being primarily functions of circuitry. Secondarily, circuitry will of course enter into any function dependent on communication over a distance. Having seen that a so-called contingent negative wave occurs in the electroencephalogram in response to expectancy (Chapter 5), it should give no cause for wonder to find electrical signs of habituation and dishabituation, the latter a response to novelty. But it may, perhaps, come as something of a surprise to find these responses recordable intracellularly in single neurons of the snail (*Aplysia*), as demonstrated in 1966 by Bruner and Tauc,[206] and elaborated by Kandel and his coworkers (1970).[205] Their findings indicate that we are dealing with one of the elementary properties of living neurons and once again show how valuable a vertical search for neurophysiological correlates can be.

Notes

1. *The Autobiography of J. J. Berzelius*, in the possession of the Royal Swedish Academy of Sciences. Quotation is from a footnote translated by the author.

2. F. Crick, *Of Molecules and Men* (Seattle: Univ. of Washington Press, 1966).

3. See several books and essays by P. Weiss, e.g., *Within the Gates of Science and Beyond* (New York: Hafner, 1971); and *Hierarchically Organized Systems* (New York: Hafner, 1971).

4. *Selected Writings of Hughlings Jackson*, ed. J. Taylor (London: Hodder and Stoughton, 1931), 2 vols.

5. P. Anderson, *New Scientist*, 2 Sept. 1971, pp. 510–513.

6. J. R. Platt, *J. Theor. Biol.* 1 (1961):342–358.

7. The 1962 Nobel Prize Lectures by F. H. C. Crick, J. D. Watson and M. H. F. Wilkins (Stockholm: Norstedt, 1963). The Prize lectures, *Nobel Lectures, Physiology or Medicine*, are available, republished in several volumes by Elsevier (Holland).

8. C. F. A. Pantin, *The Relation Between the Sciences* (Cambridge: Cambridge Univ. Press, 1968).

9. E. Mayr, *Science* 134 (1963):1501–1506. See also *Animal Species and Evolution* (Cambridge, Mass.: Harvard Univ. Press, 1963).

10. J. Monod, *Le Hasard et la Nécessité* (Paris: Editions du Seuil, 1970).

11. "Purposive behavior" has long been accepted by psychologists. See E. C. Tolman, *Purposive Behavior in Animals and Men* (New York: Appleton-Century-Crofts, 1967) (1st ed. 1932). Recent presentations include M. A. Boden, *Purposive Explanation in Psychology* (New York: Oxford Univ. Press, 1972), and D. E. Broadbent, *Behavior* (New York: Basic Books, 1961).

12. N. Barlow, ed., *The Autobiography of Charles Darwin* (London: Collins, 1958).

13. See C. D. Darlington, *Genetics and Man* (London: Allen & Unwin, 1964).

14. Consult any modern account of evolutionary theory, such as those by Mayr (note 9) or Darlington (note 13). For a special account, see W. Hovanitz, *Symp. Soc. Exp. Biol.* 7 (1953):238–251.

15. For the development of the lateral line organ, see W. A. van Bergrijk, "The evolution of vertebrate hearing," *Contributions to Sensory Physiology*, ed. W. D. Neff, vol. 2 (New York: Academic Press, 1967), pp. 1–49.

16. Nobel Prize to Sir Ronald Ross in 1902.

17. G. Edelman and R. Porter, *Les Prix Nobel en 1972*. (Stockholm: Norstedt, 1973).

18. Lady Mary Wortley Montagu's 52 Turkish Embassy letters are reviewed in *The Familiar Letter in the Eighteenth Century*, ed. H. Anderson, Ph. B. Daghlian, and I. Ehrenpreis (Lawrence: Univ. Press of Kansas, 1968), pp. 49–70.

19. K. von Frisch, *Aus dem Leben der Bienen* (Berlin, Göttingen, Heidelberg: Springer-Verlag, 1953).

20. M. Schultze, *Strickers Handbuch der Lehre von den Geweben* 2 (1871):977–1034.

21. J. W. Craik, *The Nature of Psychology: A Selection of Papers*, ed. S. L. Sherwood (Cambridge: Cambridge Univ. Press, 1966), paper no. 24.

22. For a history of retinal work, see R. Granit, *Sensory Mechanisms of the Retina* (London: Oxford Univ. Press, 1947; New York: Hafner, 1963).

23. W. Weaver, *Am. Sci.* 36 (1948):536–544.

24. C. H. Waddington, *The Strategy of the Genes* (London: Allen & Unwin, 1957); E. Mayr, "The emergence of evolutionary novelties," in *Evolution after Darwin*, vol. 1, ed. S. Tax (Chicago, Ill.: Univ. of Chicago Press, 1960); T. Dobzhansky, *Evolution, Genetics and Man* (New York: Wiley, 1967).

25. N. K. Jerne, *Sci. Am.* 229 (1973):52–60.

219   Notes

26. R. Descartes, *Discours de la Méthode* (Paris: Éditions Garnier Frères, 1950).

27. A. Brodal, "The 'wiring patterns' of the brain" in *The Neurosciences: Paths of Discovery*, ed. F. P. Worden, J. P. Swazey and G. Adelman (Cambridge, Mass.: The MIT Press, 1975), pp. 121–140.

28. See any physiological textbook; for details, see J. C. Eccles, *The Physiology of the Synapses* (Heidelberg. Springer-Verlag, 1964).

29. The subsynaptic membrane is that part of the cell membrane on which a synapse projects.

30. R. Granit, "In defense of teleology" in *Brain and Human Behavior*, ed. A. G. Karzman and J. C. Eccles (Heidelberg: Springer-Verlag, 1972), pp. 400–408.

31. G. Sommerhoff, *Analytical Biology* (New York: Oxford Univ. Press, 1950).

32. D'Arcy W. Thompson, *Growth and Form*, vol. 1 (London: Cambridge Univ. Press, 1952), p. 139.

33. J. Annett, *Feedback and Human Behavior* (Harmondsworth: Penguin, 1969).

34. N. Wiener, *Cybernetics or Control and Communication in the Animal and the Machine* (Cambridge, Mass.: The MIT Press, 2d ed., 1961).

35. E. G. T. Liddell and C. S. Sherrington, *Proc. R. Soc., B.* 96 (1924):212–242.

36. S. Ramón y Cajal, *Histologie du Système Nerveux de l'Homme et des Vertébrés* (reprinted by Instituto Ramón y Cajal, Madrid, 1952).

37. For this and other references to the literature on motor problems, see R. Granit, *The Basis of Motor Control* (New York: Academic Press, 1970).

38. The work of H. K. Hartline is conveniently available in *Studies on Excitation and Inhibition in the Retina*, ed. F. Ratliff (New York: Rockefeller Univ. Press, 1974).

39. R. W. Sperry, "Mechanisms of neural maturation" in *Handbook of Experimental Psychology*, ed. S. S. Stevens (New York: Wiley, 1951).

40. Reviews of experiments on adaptability or plasticity are found in M. Jacobson, *Developmental Neurobiology* (New York: Holt, Rinehart and Winston, 1970) and in R. M. Gaze, *The Formation of Nervous Connections* (New York: Academic Press, 1970).

41. M. Jacobson and R. K. Hunt, *Sci. Am.* 228 (1973):26–35.

42. D. H. Hubel and T. N. Wiesel, *J. Physiol. (Lond.)* 206 (1970):419–436.

43. H. V. B. Hirsch and D. N. Spinelli, *Science* 168 (1970):869–871; Blakemore and G. F. Cooper, *Nature* 228 (1970):477–478; C. Blakemore and D. E. Mitchell, *Nature* 241 (1973):467–468.

44. D. H. Hubel and T. N. Wiesel, *J. Physiol. (Lond.)* 148 (1959):574–591.

45. G. M. Stratton, *Psychol. Rev.* 4 (1897):341–360; 463–486.

46. Granit, *Receptors and Sensory Perception* (New Haven: Yale Univ. Press, 1955).

47. A. Fiorentini, C. Ghez and L. Maffei, *J. Physiol. (Lond.)* 227 (1972):313–322.

48. B. G. Cragg, *J. Anat.* 101 (1967):639–654.

49. D. A. Sholl, *The Organization of the Cerebral Cortex* (London: Methuen, 1956).

50. J. R. Marotte and R. F. Mark, *Brain Res.* 19 (1970):41–62.

51. I. Kohler, *Sitzber. Österr. Akad. Wiss.* 277 (1951) and *Sci. Am.* 206 (1962):62.

52. R. Held and A. Hein, *J. Comp. Psychol.* 56 (1963):872–876.

53. For reviews on the voluminous literature on language areas, see W. Penfield and L. Roberts, *Speech and Brain Mechanisms* (Princeton: Princeton Univ. Press, 1959); R. C. Oldfield and J. C. Marshall, eds., *Language* (Baltimore: Penguin, 1968); N. Geschwind, *Sci. Am.* 226 (1972):76–83.

54. R. W. Sperry, *Arch. Neurol. Psychiat.* 58 (1947):452–473.

55. J. H. Boyes, ed., *Bunnell's Surgery of the Hand* (Philadelphia: Lippincott, 1974).

56. E. Moberg, *Hand* 4 (1972):201–206. Also personal communication.

57. A. J. Buller, J. C. Eccles and R. M. Eccles, *J. Physiol. (Lond.)* 150 (1960):399–416.

58. M. Bárány and R. J. Close, *J. Physiol. (Lond.)* 213 (1971):455–474.

59. F. C. A. Romanul and J. P. Van Der Meulen, *Arch. Neurol.* 17 (1967):387–402.

60. For a review of axoplasmic flow, see R. J. Lasek, *Exp. Neurol.* 21 (1968):41–51.

61. For a review, see S. K. Sharpless, *Ann. Rev. Physiol.* 26 (1964):357–388; M. R. Rosenzweig, E. L. Bennett, and M. C. Diamond, *Sci. Am.* 226 (1972):22–29.

62. C. S. Sherrington, *Man on His Nature* (Cambridge: Cambridge Univ. Press, 1941).

63. B. Kurtén, *Comment Biol. Soc. Sci. Fenn.* no. 36 (1971):3–8.

64. See reviews by R. Bauchot and R. Platel, *La Recherche* 4 (1973):1069–1077; B. Rensch, *Naturwiss.* 45 (1958):145–154; 175–180; H. Stephan, "Evolution of primate brains; a comparative anatomical investigation" in *The Functional and Evolutionary Biology of Primates*, ed. R. Tuttle (Chicago: Aldine/Atherton, 1972), p. 162.

65. J. S. Beritoff, *Neural Mechanisms of Higher Vertebrate Behavior* (Boston: Little, Brown, 1965).

66. R. L. Halloway, *Brain Res.* 7 (1968):121–172.

67. Many maps of the cerebral cortex of man have been published, but because these maps cannot be based on work with a single individual, a large amount of experience is required, such as that found at Montreal Neurological Institute of McGill University. See W. Penfield and T. Rasmussen, *The Cerebral Cortex of Man* (New York: Macmillan, 1950).

68. For a general brief introduction to brain physiology and neurology, the little book by Ritchie Russell, *Brain, Memory, Learning* (Oxford: Clarendon Press, 1959), will be found useful. Interesting but highly speculative is K. H. Pribram, *Languages of the Brain* (Englewood Cliffs, N.J.: Prentice-Hall, 1971) dealing with "principles of neuropsychology"; neurophysiology is represented by J. C. Eccles, *The Understanding of the Brain* (New York: McGraw-Hill, 1973), and neuroanatomy combined with cybernetics in J. Z. Young, *A Model of the Brain* (Oxford: Clarendon Press, 1961).

69. S. A. Talbot and W. H. Marshall, *Am. J. Ophthalmol.* 24 (1941):1255–1264; P. M. Daniel and D. Whitteridge, *J. Physiol. (Lond.)* 159 (1961):203–221.

70. D. Shannon, *Neurosciences Research Symposium Summaries*, vol. 1 (Cambridge, Mass.: The MIT Press, 1966), p. 148.

71. P. Teilhard de Chardin, *Le Phénomène Humain* (Paris: Éditions du Seuil, 1955).

72. M. Polanyi, *Science* 160 (1968):1308–1312.

73. The psychologist's attitude to consciousness is well represented by Cyril Burt, *Br. J. Psychol.* 53 (1962):229–242. A standpoint reminiscent of my own is taken by R. W. Sperry in *Psychol. Rev.* 76 (1969):532–536.

74. W. James, *The Principles of Psychology*, vol. 1 (New York: Macmillan, 1891).

75. B. Libet has reviewed their work in *Brain and Conscious Experience*, ed. J. C. Eccles (Heidelberg and New York: Springer-Verlag, 1966). This book contains the papers of a Papal Symposium in which conscious awareness was most directly considered in the contributions by Moruzzi, Penfield, and Sperry.

76. K. J. W. Craik, *Br. J. Psychol.* 38 (1947–1948):56–61; 142–148; M. A. Vince, *Br. J. Psychol.* 38 (1948):149–157.

77. There is a large literature dealing with arousal, alertness, and attention. For reviews, see H. W. Magoun, *The Waking Brain* (Springfield, Ill.: Thomas, 1958); C. R. Evans and T. B. Mulholland, *Attention in Neurophysiology* (London: Butterworth, 1969); O. Pompeiano, "Reticular Formation" in *Handbook of Sensory Physiology*, vol. 2 (New York: Springer, 1973).

78. Hans Berger's discovery, its development and practical applications are well presented in F. A. and E. I. Gibbs, *Atlas of Electroencephalography* (Reading, Mass.: Addison-Wesley, 1948).

79. G. Walter's discovery of the expectancy wave or contingent negative variations in *Arch. Psychiatr. Nervenkr.* 206 (1964–1965):309–322. Walter, with several coworkers, has described recent developments in *J. Electroencephalogr. Clin. Neurophysiol.* 23 (1967):197–206. The contingent negative wave mainly involves the frontal cortex, which at the surface becomes electronegative by about 20 μv with respect to deeper structures.

80. W. Penfield, *The Excitable Cortex in Conscious Man* (Liverpool: Liverpool Univ. Press, 1958). Penfield has described "engrams" (a term used for retained information) elicitable by electrical stimulation in a large number of reviews.

81. See R. W. Sperry's recent summary in *Psychophysiology of Thinking*, ed. F. J. McGuigan and R. A. Schoonover (New York: Academic Press, 1973), the book by M. S. Gazzaniga, *The Bisected Brain* (New York: Appleton-Century-Crofts, 1970), or S. J. Diamond and J. S. Beaumont, *Hemisphere Function in the Human Brain* (London: Elek. Books, 1974).

82. There is a detailed examination of the properties of the nondominant hemisphere by J. E. Bogen in three articles under the general heading "The other side of the brain," the third with G. M. Bogen, *Bull. Los Angeles Neurol. Soc.* 34 (1969):73–105, 135–162, 191–220. The reference to Luria's work is in them.

83. W. C. Dement, *Electroencephalogr. Clin. Neurophysiol.* 10 (1958):291–296; M. Jouvet, *Physiol. Rev.* 47 (1967):117–177; O. Pompeiano, "A neural model of REM sleep" in *Sleep*, ed. W. P. Koella and P. Levin (Basel: S. Karger, 1973).

84. H. Head, *Aphasia and Kindred Disorders of Speech*, vol. 1 (New York: Hafner, 1963), p. 490.

85. G. Moruzzi, "The sleep-waking cycle," *Ergebn. Physiol.* 64 (1972):1–165.

86. D. O. Hebb's laboratory in Montreal initiated work on these lines. A critical review of the whole field of sensory deprivation by J. P. Zubeck, *Br. Med. Bull.* 20 (1964):38–42.

87. N. Tinbergen, *Proc. R. Soc., B.* 182 (1972):385–410.

88. See C. S. Sherrington, *The Endeavour of Jean Fernel* (London: Cambridge Univ. Press, 1946).

89. E. Mach, *Die Analyse der Empfindungen*, 8th ed. (Jena: Fischer, 1919), pp. 29–30.

90. A. N. Whitehead, *Modes of Thought* (New York: Capricorn Books, 1955).

91. G. T. Fechner, *Elemente der Psychophysik* (Leipzig: Breitkopf and Härtel, 1862).

92. The 1834 paper was in Latin. The results are accessible in Weber's review, "Der Tastsinn und das Gemeingefühl," *Wagners Handwörterbuch der Physiologie* 3 (1846):481–588.

93. See E. D. Adrian, *The Basis of Sensation* (London: Christophers, 1928).

94. The old psychophysical work will be found in H. Aubert, *Physiologie der Netzhaut* (Breslau: Morgenstern, 1865); H. von Helmholtz, *Handbuch der physiologischen Optik* (Leipzig: 1867); E. Hering, *Grundzüge der Lehre vom Lichtsinn*, republished in *Graefe-Saemisch Handbuch der gesamten Augenheilkunde*, 2nd ed. (1925, vol. 3, part 12, pp. 1–294); J. von Kries, "Die Gesichtsempfindungen," *Nagels Handb. Physiol.* 3 (1904):109–282; A. König, *Gesammelte Abhandlungen zur physiologischen Optik* (Leipzig: Barth, 1903).

95. W. Kühne, "Chemische Vorgänge in der Netzhaut," *Hermanns Handb. Physiol.* 3 (1879):235–342.

96. C. S. Sherrington, *The Integrative Action of the Nervous System* (New Haven: Yale Univ. Press, 1906).

97. J. J. Gibson, *The Senses Considered as Perceptual Systems* (Boston: Houghton Mifflin, 1966).

98. The trichromatic theory of color vision is generally referred to as the Young-Helmholtz color theory.

224 Notes

99. The recent literature on the retina is so enormous and progress has been so rapid, mainly because of improved microelectrodes and electronics, that it is impossible to refer to all the individual contributions. For a general orientation a good starting point is the appropriate volumes of the *Handbook of Sensory Physiology* (New York: Springer-Verlag, 1971). Some leading references have been selected for this chapter. See also note 22 (for the history of retinal electrophysiology).

100. H. B. Barlow and W. B. Levick, *J. Physiol. (Lond.)* 178 (1965):477–504.

101. S. W. Kuffler, *J. Neurophysiol.* 16 (1953):37–68.

102. A. L. Yarbus, *Eye Movements and Vision* (New York: Plenum Press, 1967).

103. The optic radiation was so named because the axons of the cells in the lateral geniculate body spread radially into the cortical visual area.

104. C. A. G. Wiersma, personal communication.

105. R. Jung, "Neuronal integration in the visual cortex and its significance for visual information," in *Sensory Communication*, ed. W. A. Rosenblith (Cambridge, Mass.: The MIT Press, 1961).

106. See note 44 for Hubel and Wiesel's early observation on cells in the visual cortex (area 17). Recent papers include *J. Physiol. (Lond.)* 195 (1968):215–243. In the papers in *J. Comp. Neurol.* 146 (1972):421–450; 158 (1974):267–294 will be found references to their work before that year (1974).

107. P. O. Bishop, J. S. Coombs and G. H. Henry, *J. Physiol. (Lond.)* 219 (1971):625–657; 231 (1973):31–60.

108. Anatomically the columnar organization of the cortex was described by Ramón y Cajal (note 36) and by Lorente de Nó in the section on cortical histology in J. F. Fulton's *Physiology of the Nervous System* (New York: Oxford Univ. Press, 1949). The first functional identification was by V. Mountcastle and T. P. S. Powell, *Bull. Johns Hopkins Hosp.* 105 (1959):173–200.

109. The development of the work on contrast and spatial frequency can be traced with the aid of the following papers all published in *J. Physiol. (Lond.)*: F. W. Campbell, B. G. Cleland, E. F. Cooper, and C. Enroth-Cugell, 198 (1968):239–251; F. W. Campbell and J. G. Robson, 197 (1968):551–556; F. W. Campbell and J. J. Kulikowski, 187 (1966):437–445; C. Blakemore and F. W. Campbell, 203 (1969):237–260; F. W. Campbell and L. Maffei, 207 (1970):635–652. See also L. Maffei and A. Fiorentini, *Vision Res.* 13 (1973):1255–1267.

225 Notes

110. L. Maffei and A. Fiorentini, *Science* 186 (1974):447–449.

111. Spatial frequency channels are interpreted in Campbell and Robson (note 109, 1968) and Blakemore and Campbell (note 109, 1969); see also L. Maffei and A. Fiorentini, *Nature* 240 (1972):479–481.

112. I. Rock, "Perception from the standpoint of psychology," *Res. Publ. Assoc. Res. Nerv. Ment. Dis.* 48 (1970):1–11.

113. The distinction between fast, phasic (transient) Y cells and more slowly and tonically responding (sustained) X cells was first noted by C. Enroth-Cugell and J. G. Robson, *J. Physiol. (Lond.)* 187 (1966):517–552, in single optic nerve fibers (cat). For further development of the role of conduction velocity of afferent fibers from retinal ganglion cells, see K.-P. Hoffman and J. Stone, *Brain Res.* 32 (1971):460–466; Stone and Hoffman, *Brain Res.* 43 (1972):610–616.

114. Experiments on selective visual deprivation, initiated by Hubel and Wiesel, are reviewed by L. Ganz, "The role of selective receptive fields in visual perception," *Res. Publ. Assoc. Res. Nerv. Ment. Dis.* 48 (1970):186–192; L. Gyllensten, T. Malmfors, and M.-L. Norrlin, *J. Comp. Neurol.* 124 (1965):149–160. The physiological abnormalities found in upper visual stations occur in spite of virtually normal retinae, as reported by S. M. Sherman and J. Stone, *Brain Res.* 60 (1973):224–230.

115. The analysis of stereopsis in single cortical cells is reviewed by J. D. Pettigrew, *Sci. Am.* 227 (1972):84–93. Some special papers are: H. B. Barlow, C. Blakemore, and J. D. Pettigrew, *J. Physiol. (Lond.)* 193 (1967):327–342; C. Blakemore, A. Fiorentini, and L. Maffei, *J. Physiol. (Lond.)* 226 (1972):725–749. The recent discoveries of Hubel and Wiesel (note 106) on ocular dominance columns are of importance for stereoscopic vision, as indicated in the text. A brief orientation in the problem of psychological cues is found in R. L. Gregory, *Nature* 207 (1965):16–19. For dependence on spatial frequency, see A. Fiorentini and L. Maffei, *Vision Res.* 11 (1971):1299–1305.

116. M. B. Bender and S. P. Diamond, *Res. Publ. Assoc. Res. Nerv. Ment. Dis.* 48 (1970):176–185. This publication contains several articles devoted to perception and its disorders. Distortions of visual perceptions are often caused by disturbed interaction between different senses. An extensive literature deals with the phenomenology of visual perception; see R. N. Haler, ed. *Contemporary Theory and Research in Visual Perception* (New York: Holt, Rinehart and Winston, 1968).

117. L. A. Riggs, F. Ratliff, J. C. Cornsweet, and T. N. Cornsweet, *J. Opt. Soc. Am.* 43 (1953):495–501; R. W. Ditchburn, *Opt. Acta* 1 (1955):171–176.

118. R. H. Wurtz, *J. Neurophysiol.* 32 (1969):975–986, 987–994.

119. S. Cooper and P. M. Daniel, *Brain* 72 (1949):1–24.

120. A. A. Skavenski, *Vision Res.* 12 (1971):221–229.

121. A good introduction to problems concerning visual illusions in R. L. Gregory, *Proc. R. Soc., B.* 171 (1968):279–296.

122. Size constancy is influenced by brain lesions. See the literature in M. Wyke, *J. Neurol. Neurosurg. Psychiatry* 23 (1960):253–261. Note that changes in size constancy occur in the absence of deficits in the primary visual afferent system.

123. R. W. Doty reviews nonstriate vision in the *Handbook of Sensory Physiology*, VII/3 (1973):483–502. See also J. W. Sprague, C. Berlucchi, and G. Rizzolatti, ibid., pp. 27–102; L. Weiskrantz, *Proc. R. Soc. B.*, 182 (1972):427–455; T. Pasik and P. Pasik, *Brain Res.* 56 (1973):165–182; *J. Neurophysiol.* 36 (1973):450–457.

124. T. Reuter and K. Virtanen, *Nature* 239 (1972):260.

125. E. J. McNichol, Jr., and G. Svaetichin, *Am. J. Ophthalmol.* 46 (1958):26–46.

126. S. M. Zeki, *Brain Res.* 53 (1973):422–427.

127. R. L. D. Valois, C. J. Smith, S. T. Kitai, and A. J. Karoly, *Science* 127 (1958):238–239. The problem of color coding is too vast for the format of this book.

128. M. Mishkin and K. H. Pribram, *J. Comp. Physiol. Psychol.* 47 (1954):14–20; for developments, see also A. Cowey and L. Weiskrantz, *Quart. J. Exp. Psychol.* 19 (1967):246–253; C. G. Gross, C. E. Rocha-Miranda, and D. B. Bender, *J. Neurophysiol.* 35 (1972):96–111; S. M. Zeki, *Brain Res.* 19 (1970):63–75.

129. See the remarks on Sherrington and Ramón y Cajal in R. Granit, *Charles Scott Sherrington: An appraisal*, British Men of Science (London: Nelson, 1966); Judith P. Swazey, *Reflexes and Motor Integration: Sherrington's Concept of Integrative Action* (Cambridge, Mass.: Harvard Univ. Press, 1969). For a general introduction to reflexology, see E. G. T. Liddell, *The Discovery of Reflexes* (Oxford: Clarendon Press, 1960).

130. A. Fick, *Mechanische Arbeit und Wärmeentwicklung bei der Muskelthätigkeit* (Leipzig: Brockhaus, 1882).

131. See R. S. Creed, D. Denny-Brown, J. C. Eccles, E. G. T. Liddell, and C. S. Sherrington, *Reflex Activity of the Spinal Cord* (Oxford: Clarendon Press, 1932).

227 Notes

132. D. Denny-Brown, *Proc. R. Soc., B.* 104 (1929):252–301; E. D. Adrian and D. W. Bronk, *J. Physiol. (Lond.)* 67 (1929):119–151; E. D. Adrian and Y. Zotterman, *J. Physiol. (Lond.)* 61 (1926):151–171; 465–483.

133. W. H. Gaskell, *J. Physiol. (Lond.)* 8 (1887):404–414.

134. A. L. Hodgkin, *The Conduction of the Nervous Impulse* (Liverpool: Liverpool Univ. Press, 1967).

135. The history of chemical and electrical theories of synaptic excitation is discussed briefly in Granit (note 129) and in greater detail in Eccles (note 28).

136. Discoveries of Dale and Loewi in *Les Prix Nobel en 1936* (Stockholm: Norstedt, 1937).

137. B. Katz, *The Release of Neural Transmitter Substances* (Liverpool: Liverpool Univ. Press, 1969); U. S. von Euler, *Noradrenaline* (Springfield, Ill.: Thomas, 1956); E. D. P. De Robertis, *Histophysiology of Synapses and Neurosecretion* (London: Pergamon Press, 1964).

138. R. Lorente de Nó, *J. Neurophysiol.* 1 (1938):187–194.

139. A. Forbes, *Physiol. Rev.* 2 (1922):361–414.

140. O. Eränkö, *Acta Endocrinol.* 18 (1955):174–179; B. Falck and N. -Å. Hillarp, *Acta Anat.* 38 (1959):277–279.

141. P. Hoffman, *Untersuchungen über die Eigenreflexe (Sehnenreflexe) menschlicher Muskeln* (Berlin: Springer, 1922); D. P. C. Lloyd, *J. Neurophysiol.* 6 (1943):293–314, 317–326.

142. J. E. Dowling and B. B. Boycott, *Proc. R. Soc., B.*, 166 (1966):80–111; T. Tomita, *Handbook of Sensory Physiology*, VII/2 (New York: Springer, 1972), pp. 483–511; A. Kaneko, J. Exp. Biol., 48 (1968):545–567.

143. L. Leksell, *Acta Physiol. Scand.* (1945):Suppl. 31.

144. K. -E. Hagbarth and Å. B. Vallbo, *Exp. Neurol.* 22 (1968):674–694; *Acta Physiol. Scand.* 76 (1969):321–334; I. Wallin, A. Hongell, and K. -E. Hagbarth, "Recordings from muscle afferents in Parkinsonian rigidity" in *New Developments in Electromyography and Clinical Neurophysiology*, ed. J. E. Desmedt (Basel: Karger, 1973), vol. 3, pp. 263–275.

145. G. Rossi, *Arch. Fisiol.* 25 (1927):146–157.

146. Load compensation is demonstrated by M. Corda, G. Eklund, and C. von Euler, *Acta Physiol. Scand.* 63 (1965):391–400; T. A. Sears, "Investigations on respiratory motoneurones of the spinal cord" in *Physiology of the Spinal Cord*, ed. J. C. Eccles and J. P. Schadé (Amsterdam: Elsevier, 1964), pp. 259–293.

147. P. B. C. Matthews, *Mammalian Muscle Receptors and Their Central Actions* (London: Arnold, 1972).

148. For details of spindle anatomy, see D. Barker, "The morphology of muscle receptors" in *Handbook of Sensory Physiology*, III/2, pp. 1–190; I. A. Boyd, *Philos. Trans. Roy. Soc.* 245 (1962):81–136; D. Barker, F. Emonet-Dénand, Y. Laporte, U. Proske, and M. J. Stacey, *J. Physiol. (Lond.)* 230 (1973):405–427.

149. C. G. Phillips, Hughlings Jackson Lecture, *Proc. Roy. Soc. Med.* 66 (1973):987–1002. Quotation from manuscript.

150. R. E. Burke, W. Z. Rymer, and J. V. Walsh, Jr., "Functional specialization in the motor unit population of cat medial gastrocnemius muscle," in *Control of Posture and Locomotion*, ed. R. B. Stein, K. G. Pearson, R. S. Smith, and J. B. Redford (New York: Plenum Press, 1973), pp. 29–43.

151. D. Denny-Brown's results in R. S. Creed et al. (note 131).

152. R. W. Doty, "Neural organization of deglutition" in *Handbook of Physiology*, Sect. 6, Vol. 4, ed. C. F. Code and W. Heidel (Baltimore: Williams and Wilkins, 1968).

153. G. B. Duchenne, *Physiologie des Mouvements* (Paris: Ballière et Fils, 1867); *Physiology of Motion*, transl. E. B. Kaplan (Philadelphia: Lippincott, 1949).

154. J. V. Basmajian, *Muscles Alive: Their Function Revealed by Electromyography* (Baltimore: Williams and Wilkins, 1962); first results by V. F. Harrison and O. A. Mortensen, *Anat. Rec.* 144 (1962):109–116.

155. A. Lundberg, "Integration in reflex pathways," in *Muscular Afferents and Motor Control, Nobel Symposium No. 1*, ed. R. Granit (Stockholm: Almqvist & Wiksell, 1966), pp. 275–305; A. I. Shapovalov, *Rev. Physiol. Biochem. Pharmacol.* 72 (1975):1–54.

156. F. B. Severin, M. L. Shik, and G. N. Orlovskij, *Biofizika* 12 (1967):502–511; 660–668.

157. C. A. G. Wiersma, *J. Neurophysiol.* 10 (1947):23–38; see also Wiersma and K. Ikeda, *Comp. Biochem. Physiol.* 12 (1964):509–525; W. J. Davis and D. Kennedy, *J. Neurophysiol.* 35 (1972):1–12, 13–19, 20–29.

158. H. H. Kornhuber and L. Deecke, *Pflüg. Arch. Ges. Physiol.* 281 (1964):52; and recent summary of the findings in this field, "Event-related slow potentials of the brain: Their relation to behaviour," ed. W. C. McCallum and J. R. Knott, *Electroencephalogr. Clin. Neurophysiol.* (1973):Suppl. 33.

229 Notes

159. H. G. Vaughan, Jr., E. G. Gross, and J. Bossom, *Exp. Neurol.* 26 (1970):253–262.

160. J. Requin and J. Paillard, *Proc. Internat. Symp. Bulg. Acad. Sci.* (1969):391–396.

161. C. G. Bernhard and E. Bohm, *Arch. Neurol. Psychiat.* 72 (1954):473–502; C. G. Phillips, "The Ferrier Lecture," *Proc. R. Soc., B.* 173 (1969):141–174.

162. D. Denny-Brown, *The Cerebral Control of Movement* (Liverpool: Liverpool Univ. Press, 1966), p. 207.

163. G. Fritsch and E. Hitzig, *Arch. Anat. Physiol.* 37 (1870):300–302.

164. D. Albe-Fessard and J. Liebeskind, *Exp. Brain Res.* 1 (1966):127–146; P. Buser and M. Imbert, "Sensory projections to the motor cortex in cats: A microelectrode study," in *Sensory Communication*, ed. W. A. Rosenblith (Cambridge, Mass.: The MIT Press, 1961), pp. 607–626.

165. L. D. Harmon, *The Neurosciences: Second Study Program*, ed. F. O. Schmitt (New York: Rockefeller Univ. Press, 1970), pp. 486–494.

166. E. V. Evarts, "Representation of movements and muscles by pyramidal tract neurons of the precentral motor cortex," in *Neurophysiological Basis of Normal and Abnormal Motor Activities*, ed. M. D. Yahr and D. Purpura (Hewlett, N. Y.: Raven Press, 1967), pp. 215–251.

167. J. C. Eccles, M. Ito, and Y. Szentágothai, *The Cerebellum as a Neural Machine* (Berlin: Springer-Verlag, 1967).

168. R. Llinás, *The Neurosciences: Second Study Program*, ed. F. O. Schmitt (New York: Rockefeller Univ. Press, 1970).

169. W. B. Scoville and B. Milner, *J. Neurol. Neurosurg. Psychiatry* 20 (1957):11–21; H.-L. Teuber, "Perception" in *Handbook of Physiology*, ed. J. Field, H. W. Magoun, and V. E. Hall, Vol. 3, Ch. 15 (Baltimore: Williams and Wilkins, 1967), pp. 1595–1668.

170. M. I. Posner, *J. Exp. Psychol.* 75 (1967):103–107.

171. P. Schilder, *The Image and Appearance of the Human Body* (New York: International Univ. Press, 1950). See also note 175.

172. F. A. Miles and J. H. Fuller, *Science* 189 (1975):1000–1002.

173. S. Bouisset and F. Lestienne, *Brain Res.* 71 (1974):451–457.

174. M. R. DeLong and P. L. Strick, *Brain Res.* 71 (1974):327–335; B. Conrad and V. B. Brooks, *J. Neurophysiol.* 37 (1974):792–804.

175. McDonald Critchley, *The Parietal Lobes* (London: Arnold, 1953).

176. The work of Mountcastle and his colleagues, *J. Neurophysiol.* 38 (1975):871–908, is well and briefly summarized by V. Mountcastle, *Johns Hopkins Med. J.* 136 (1975):109–131. See J. Hyvärinen and A. Poranen, *Brain* 97 (1974):673–692.

177. R. Held and A. Hein, "A neural model for labile sensorimotor coordinations," in *Biological Prototypes and Sensorimotor Coordinations*, vol.1, ed. E. E. Bernard and M. R. Kare (New York: Plenum Press, 1962), pp. 71–74.

178. K. S. Lashley, *Am. J. Physiol.* 43 (1917):169–194.

179. Observations mentioned by K. -E. Hagbarth on p. 16 in report of a conference on the control of movement and posture, summarized by R. Granit and R. E. Burke, *Brain Res.* 53 (1973):1–28.

180. J. Olds and P. Milner, *J. Comp. Physiol. Psychol.* 47 (1954):419–427, and *The Role of Pleasure in Behavior*, ed. R. G. Heath (London, 1964).

181. See C. R. Evans and T. B. Mulholland, *Attention in Neurophysiology* (London: Butterworth, 1969).

182. D. R. Humphrey, E. M. Schmidt, and W. D. Thompson, *Science* 170 (1970):758–762.

183. C. Taylor, "The explanation of purposive behaviour" in *Explanation in the Behavioural Sciences*, ed. R. Borger and F. Coffi (London: Cambridge Univ. Press, 1970).

184. A. G. Feldman and G. N. Orlovsky, *Brain Res.* 84 (1975):181–194.

185. Ewald Hering's article, based largely on the work of his pupil Joseph Breuer, is referred to in a historical account by Elisabeth Ullmann in *Breathing: Hering-Breuer Centenary Symposium*, ed. for the Ciba Foundation by R. Porter (London: J & A Churchill, 1970), pp. 1–15, in a discussion of early physiological contributions to the idea of feedback control.

186. W. B. Cannon proposed the term "homeostatics" in a jubilee volume for Charles Richet (1926) and altered it to "homeostasis" in an article in *Res. Publ. Assoc. Res. Nerv. Ment. Dis.* (1930), pp. 181–198.

187. For further information on cybernetics in biology, see K. E. Machin, "Feedback theory and its application to biological systems," *Symp. Soc. Exp. Biol.* 18 (1964):421–446; D. McKay, *Information, Mechanism and Meaning* (Cambridge, Mass.: The MIT Press, 1969).

188. L. Stark, *Neurological Control Systems: Studies in Bioengineering* (New York: Plenum Press, 1968).

189. K. S. Lashley, *Brain Mechanisms and Intelligence* (Chicago: Chicago Univ. Press, 1930).

231 Notes

190. R. Galambos, T. T. Norton, and G. P. Frommer, *Exp. Neurol.* 18 (1967):8–25.

191. Broca's and Wernicke's classical findings are often reviewed. See F. L. Darley, ed., *Brain Mechanisms Underlying Speech and Language* (New York: Grune & Stratton, 1967) and the discussion in Chapter 3.

192. See the discussion of arousal in Chapter 5 and note 77.

193. K. H. Pribram and D. McGuinness, "Arousal, activation and effort in the control of attention," *Psychol. Rev.* 82 (1975):116–149.

194. From the vast literature on memory some selected introductions are: O. L. Zangwill, *Br. Med. Bull.* 20 (1964):43–48; I. S. Russell, *Br. Med. Bull.* 27 (1971):278–285; D. E. Broadbent, *Proc. R. Soc., B.*, 175 (1970):333–350; W. J. H. Nauta, "Some brain structures and functions related to memory," *Neurosci. Res. Symposium, Summaries*, vol. 1 (Cambridge, Mass.: The MIT Press, 1966); C. Symmonds, *Brain* 89 (1966):624–644; G. A. Talland and N. C. Waugh, ed., *The Pathology of Memory* (New York: Academic Press, 1969); S. Bogoch, *The Biochemistry of Memory* (New York: Oxford Univ. Press, 1968); F. R. John, *Mechanisms of Memory* (New York: Academic Press, 1970).

195. D. Zeidel and R. W. Sperry, *Brain* 97 (1974):263–272.

196. B. Milner, *Neuropsychologia*, 6 (1968):175–179, 191–209. Also note 169.

197. L. Weiskrantz, *Proc. R. Soc. B.*, 171 (1968):335–352.

198. U. Ungerstedt, *Acta Physiol. Scand.* (1971):Suppl. 367.

199. For historical notes on the L-DOPA cure, see O. Hornykiewicz, "Parkinson's disease: From brain homogenate to treatment," *Fed. Proc.* 32 (1973):183–190; A. Barbeau and F. H. McDowell, ed., *L-DOPA and Parkinsonism* (Philadelphia: Davis, 1970).

200. J. Altman and W. J. Anderson, *J. Comp. Neurol.* 146 (1972):355–405.

201. Description of Setchenow's experiment on p. 40 in R. Granit, *Charles Scott Sherrington: An Appraisal* (London: Nelson, 1966).

202. See K. S. Cole, *Membranes, Ions and Impulses* (Berkeley: Univ. of California Press, 1968); A. L. Hodgkin and A. F. Huxley, *J. Physiol. (Lond.)* 117 (1952):500–544. See also note 134.

203. F. A. Dodge and B. Frankenhaeuser, *J. Physiol. (Lond.)* 143 (1958):76–90.

204. M. J. Cohen, *Comp. Biochem. Physiol.* 8 (1963):223–243.

205. A. Arvanitaki, *J. Neurophysiol.* 5 (1942):89–108, started such work at

this early date. L. Tauc, *Arch. Ital. Biol.* 96 (1958):78–110; E. R. Kandel et al., *Science* 167 (1970):1740–1748, and *Sci. Am.* 223 (1970):57. See also note 157 for work on the crayfish.

206. The late R. Hernandez-Peón devoted much experimental work to such problems; for example, see A. Davidovich and M. Miranda in *Acta Neurol. Latinoamer.* 8 (1962):180–186, but the interest is focused on single cells of *Aplysia* by J. Bruner and L. Tauc, *Nature* 210 (1966):37–39, work continued and expanded by Kandel and his coworkers (note 205).

Name Index

Adrian, E. D., 87, 139, 223n93, 227n132
Albe-Fessard, D., 170, 229n164
Altman, J., 209, 231n200
Anderson, P., 5, 217n5
Anderson, W. J., 209, 231n200
Annett, J., 31, 219n33
Arvanitaki, A., 212, 231n205
Aubert, H., 92, 223n94

Bárány, M., 46, 220n58
Barker, D., 153, 228n148
Barlow, H. B., 100, 120, 224n100, 225n115
Basmajian, J. V., 161, 228n154
Bauchot, R., 221n64
Beaumont, J. S., 222n81
Behring, E. A. von, 14
Bender, D. B., 226n128
Bender, M. B., 123, 225n116
Bennett, E. L., 220n61
Berger, H., 28, 78, 222n78
Bergrijk, W. A. van, 218n15
Beritoff, J. S., 55, 221n65

Berlucchi, C., 226n123
Bernard, C., 197
Bernhard, C. G., 168, 229n161
Berzelius, J., 1, 9, 19, 74, 126, 217n1
Betz, V. A., 173
Bishop, P. O., 108, 224n107
Blakemore, C., 38, 39, 112, 114, 115, 117, 120, 121, 220n43, 224n109, 225n115
Boden, M. A., 218n11
Bogen, G. M., 222n82
Bogen, J. E., 82, 222n82
Bogoch, S., 231n194
Bohm, E., 168, 229n161
Bohr, N., 71, 72
Boll, F., 19
Bossom, J., 165, 229n159
Bouisset, S., 181, 229n173
Boycott, B. B., 145, 227n142
Boyd, I. A., 153, 228n148
Breuer, J., 230n185
Broadbent, D. E., 204, 205, 218n11, 231n194

234   Name Index

237 Name Index

Subject Index

243 Subject Index

189, 202, 203. *See also* "Demand"
Psychophysical parallelism, 19
Psychophysics. *See also* Visual contrast, Vision
classical aspects of, 88–92
modern version of, defined, 94
Pulfrich effect, 126, 128
Purposiveness, 6–10, 25, 29, 30,
34, 36, 37, 41, 47, 49, 96, 128,
129, 135, 158, 161, 164, 175,
176, 187, 192, 201
Pyramidal tract. *See also* Motor
area
origin of, 169, 170
sensory projections of, 170, 171
size in different animals, 52

Reaction time, 77
"Readiness potential." *See* Voluntary movement
Reciprocal innervation, 144, 163,
174, 193–196
Recurrent fibers, 32, 33, 193–195.
See also Inhibition, recurrent
"Reductionism," 5, 85, 210
Redundancy, 66–68, 198, 201
Reflexes, 136–145
conditioned, 28, 36, 37
interaction of, 137, 138, 193–196
monosynaptic, 144, 145, 160,
173, 195
postural, 134, 151, 198, 213
reciprocal (*see* Reciprocal innervation)
scratch, 30
stretch, 32, 144, 146–154, 163,
198
Release, 149, 206–209
Resonance
acoustic, 92
visual (*see* Visual contrast)

Reticular activating system, 79
Retina, 18–20, 33, 62, 96–101,
112
color contrast in, 130
directional cells in, 52, 97, 100
inhibition in, 33, 97, 98
on-off discharges from, 98, 99,
104
receptive fields of, 100, 101, 104
Rhodopsin, 19, 91

Sensory deprivation, 83, 84
Serendipity in Nature, 10, 11
Servomechanisms, 31, 152–154
Sleep, 62, 73, 78, 79, 150, 202,
203
paradoxical or REM, 82
Somatotopic connections, 27
Sound localization, 92
Specificity, 21, 37, 43, 44, 143,
201, 204
Spectral distribution of sensitivity,
90, 91
Speech, 43, 56, 61, 63, 68, 69,
202, 213
Split-brain patients, 68, 80–82,
202, 205. *See also* Brain
Spontaneous activity of cells, 27,
67, 105
Stabilization of performance, 32,
194, 196, 211
Stabilized images on retina, 102,
124
Stereoscopic vision, 119–122
Striate cortex, 104
Swallowing, 161, 164
Synapses, 5, 24, 27, 41, 46, 48,
92, 138, 142, 143
term defined, 136
Synaptic transmission, 141, 142.
See also Transmitters
Systems analyzed. *See* Organizations